ROLE (

(CLALASS –I & II)AND INNFECTIONS

By
Varsha Bhagvatprasad Trivedi

Abstract

Chronic kidney disease is iceberg in the world, particularly in developing countries. Progressive chronic kidney disease leads to end-stage renal disease. The end-stage renal disease occurs when the kidneys are no longer able to function at a level that is necessary for day-to-day life. Either dialysis or kidney transplant is the mode of treatment. There is an acute need to increase kidney transplant to offer a better life to end-stage renal disease patients. Access to dialysis and kidney transplant in the developing world is limited because of a shortage of organ, affordability and very expensive treatment for a lifetime. Hence, optimizing renal allograft survival is essential. Health care between urban and rural populations is different due to disparities in wealth and literacy. The most common causes of kidney disease in India in both men and women are diabetes and hypertension. This study aimed to evaluate clinical outcomes and identify poor prognostic factors in the renal transplant at the institute of kidney diseases and research center (IKDRC), Ahmedabad. Antibody-mediated and viral infections lead to rejection. The rationale of the present study was to understand the different mechanisms involved in the molecular pathways of rejections. The study was designed with two main objectives in mind to understand the causes of rejections in spite of best HLA matching. Also, there is a need to address problems involved in kidney transplants like morbidity, rejections, infections and long term survival of the graft

1) To correlate the presence of class-I and class-II antibodies with rejection episodes.

2) To correlate viral infection with rejections.

It has been pointed out that the presence of donor-specific antibodies (DSA) in ESRD cases are seen in high-risk patients. Inadequate immunosuppression and non-adherence lead to graft rejection. *Denovo* DSAs are predominantly directed to donor HLA (human leukocyte antigen) class II mismatches and usually occur during the first year of a kidney transplant, but they can appear anytime, even after several years.

To achieve the above objectives the study was planned to monitor pre and post-transplant patients included in our study. Different tests were used to know the immunological status of the patient in the pre and post-transplant period. HLA Typing of patient and donor to know there HLA antigens and matching. Complement mediated Lymphocyte cross-matching for detection of auto and donor-specific IgM and IgG cytotoxic antibody. Flow cytometry cross matches for detection of IgG donor-specific antibodies against T & B cells. The third test used was HLA antibody specificity and titer detection by the Luminex platform. All three test is carried out before the transplant. If the screening test was positive then single antigen bead test was advised. These tests were also used in post-transplant monitoring for HLA DSA antibody. Presence of DSA HLA antibody leads to rejection and then graft lost if not treated. Testing of infections like viral, bacterial and fungal was carried out as and when required in pre and post-transplant period. Culture and sensitivity for bacterial and fungal infections and for viral infection detection real-time PCR techniques used.

Our study it has been shown that DQ antibodies are associated with significantly reduced graft survival. Importantly, antibody-mediated rejection and graft loss did not occur in patients with low levels of DQ-only antibodies. This report details the DQ DSA incidence and actual 5-year post graft outcomes. The mean serum creatinine and proteinuria were significantly higher in patients who developed HLA-DQ antibodies. The 5-year graft survival was significantly worse when HLA-DQ antibodies were combined with non-DQ antibodies. This study found that donor-specific HLA-DQ antibodies were the most common type detected and these antibodies may contribute to inferior graft outcomes. Overall antibody-mediated rejections are an important aspect to deal under the organ transplant outcome. Along with the presence of HLA antibodies, other important causes of rejection are viral infections like CMV (4.5%), BKV (3.7%) HBsAg (1.8%), HCV (3.7%), Ebstain-Bar viruses' leads to immunomodulation followed rejection.

Acknowledgements

It is a privilege on my behalf to thank the people who made this thesis possible. When I introspect, I feel that it would have been impossible for me to finish this work without the combined effort of my teachers, friends, fellow colleagues and grace of god. Hence,Iwant to pay my sincere gratitude from the bottom of my heart to all who were associated during the completion of this work.

I express my sincere gratitude to the Nirma University for allowing me to join Ph.D. Programme and providing support during the course of this programme. I am thankful to Dr Karsanbhai K. Patel (President, NirmaUniversity), Shri K.K. Patel (VicePresident), Dr.AnupK. Singh(Director General), Shri D.P.Chhaya (A&GA), Dr.A.S.Patel (Dy.Registrar),Dr. Dhaval Pujara(Dean,FDSR), Ms. A.P. Prashyaand Mr. Sachin Kikani.

I am deeply thankful to my guide Dr.Sarat Dalai, for accepting me as a student, for his guidance and constructive approach. His inputs to thework, commitment to highest standards have motivated me and incorporation of which has helped in my scientific perception for the better. I remain thankful for his insightful suggestions and encouragement throughout my study. I am very much thankful to him for taking effort in reading the draft of this thesis and providing me with valuable suggestions to improve the thesis.

I humbly thankful to Dr.H L Trivedi for guiding me and giving me permission to do my further study also allowing me to use well-established laboratory set up to carry out my research at Institute of kidney diseases and research Center on renal transplantation. Academic activity at IKDRC and ITS has help me in exchanging lot of ideas with peers and moreover furnishing my presentation skills. I am also thankful to our director Dr. V.V Mishra for his support.

I would like to extend my sincere gratitude to Professor Suraksha Agrawal, for her perceptive advice and guidance from the very first day of my research work and for providing me with valuable inputs due to her long scientific experience. She has been encouraging force in the growth as a researcher. I am grateful to her for being able to finish this work, constant encouragement and personal guidance which have provided a main stay foundation in the

Completion of my thesis. Her wide knowledge and logical way of thinking have been of great value for me. Shehas always challenged me to set a higher bar and to look for solutions to difficult problems. She mirrored back my ideas so that I was able to hear them aloud that helped to shape my thesis work.

I am also thankful to Dr. Sunil Trivedi for his constant support and motivation throughout the work of this thesis. His extensive discussions around basics of science and interesting explorations have been very helpful. I also owe him for making me understand many statistical applications.

I gratefully acknowledge the support of Dr.Susan Saidman throughout my thesis writing she provided encouragement, sound advice good teaching friendly behavior and lots of good ideas.

I cannot say an enough thank you gratefully acknowledge the support of Professors of nephrology department for providing me with the samples and valuable clinical information imperative for my study.

I am also thankful to Dr.Sonal Baxi and all faculty members of institute of science for their guidance throughout my work.

I am appreciative to my staff members for providing a stimulating environment in which I was able to learn and grow. I wish to extend my heartiest thanks to all those who have helped me with my work. Mr.Ketan,Mrs.Jaysharee, Mrs. Anila, Mrs. Sunita, Ms. Mira, Mrs. Khushbu, Ms. Priti.

I am also thankful to the computer department staff members Mr.Yezdi, Mr.Tarun and Mr.Sanjay

I am also thankful to Mrs.Suhanee, Mr. Paresh, Mrs. Annal for their guidance in various statistical analyses, and for his essential assistance in rectifying mistakes and making me understand the statistical analysis. Related to my work. Moreover, I am extremely thankful for his patience and for the valuable time that he has spent during my data analysis. Special thanks to Librarian for his patience and sincere efforts to make this thesis absolutely plagiarism free.

I acknowledge the help extended by administrative office staff members I came across at the Nirma University and institute of kidney diseases & research center Mr.Devang, Mr.Hasit,

Mr.partha, Mr.Kamal,Ms. Nalini, Librarian Ms. Jyotsna For their help pertaining to various administrative works.

All of you have always showered me with their inspiring words and motivated to achieve my goal. I will be always thankful to them for being my well-wishers and the source of inspiration throughout my work.

I would like to thank all the patients and their donors who co-operated in giving blood samples for this study. Lastly, I have ensured to pay my gratitude to all those who are associated with the accomplishment of this work but if I missed anyone, please accept my apology as it is totally unintentional.

Content

List of Tables

List of Charts

List of Figures

Abbreviations, Notations & Nomenclatures

μ: micro

μL: microliter

Å: Angstrom

AHG: Anti human globulin

AMR or AbMR: Antibody mediated rejection

ADCC-Antibody dependent cell mediated cytotoxicity

APC: Antigen presenting cell

A: Adenine

BKV: BK virus

BKVAN: BK virus associated nephropathy

C: Cytosine

CD: Cluster of differentiation

CDC: Complement dependent cytotoxicity

CGN: Chronic Glomerulonephritis

CIN: Chronic Interstitial Nephritis

CKD: Chronic Kidney Disease

CNIS: Calcineurin inhibitors

CRF-chronic renal failure

CRP-C-reactive protein

CTL: Cytotoxic T lymphocytes

CVD: Cardiovascular Disease

CMV: Cytomegalo virus

DTT: Dithiothreitol

DSA: Donor specific antibody

ddH2O: double-distilled autoclaved water

ddNTP: Dideoxynucleotides tri-phosphate

DN: Diabetic Nephropathy

dnDSA: Denovo donor specific antibody

dNTP: Dinucleotide tri-phosphate

EDTA: Ethylene diamine tetra acetic acid

ESRD: End stage renal disease

EtBr: Ethidium Bromide

EBV: Epstein bar virus

eGFR- Estimated glomerular filteration rate

ECM-Extra cellular matrix

FCM: Flow crossmatch

G: Guanine

GCKR: Glucokinase (Hexokinase 4) Regulator

GFR: Glomerular Filtration Rate

HAART: Highly active antiretroviral therapy

HD: Hemodialysis

HIV: Human immune deficiency virus

HLA: Human leukocyte antigens

HLAab: HLA antibodies

HPLC: High performance liquid chromatography

HTN: Hypertension

HGFIN-Hematopoietic growth factor inducible neurokian-1

HWE: Hardy-Wienberg Equilibrum

HBV: Hepatitis B virus

HBsAg: Hepatitis B surface antigen.

ICAM: Intracellular adhesion molecule

IKDRC: Institute of Kidney Disease and Research Center

IL: Interleukin

IPD: Immuno Polymorphism Database

IRI: Ischemia-reperfusion injury

ITAM: Immune receptor tyrosine based activating molecules

ITIM: Immune receptor tyrosine based inhibitory molecules

IMPDH: Inosine-5 monophosphate dehydrogenase

KARAP: Killer cell activating receptor associated protein

KIR: Killer immunoglobulin like receptor

LAIR: Leukocyte-associated inhibitory receptor

LD: Linkage disequilibrium

LILR: Leukocyte immunoglobulin like receptor

LRC: Leukocyte receptor complex

MHC: Major histocompatibility complex

mM: Milli Molar

MMP20: Matrix Metallopeptidase 20

MFI: Mean fluorescence intensity

MMPED2: Metallophosphoesterase Domain Containing 2

NK cell: Natural killer cell

NF: Nuclear Factor

NFAT: Nuclear Factor of Activated T cell

OD: Optical Density

PAMP: Pathogen associated molecular patterns

PCA: Principal component analysis

PCR: Polymerase chain reaction

pM: Pico mole

Pmp: Per million population

PTLD: Post transplant lymphoproliferative disorder

RA: Rheumatoid arthritis

RCLB: Red cell lysis buffer

REML: Restricted maximum likelihood

RF: Renal failure

RT: Room temperature

SA: Single antigen.

SBT: Sequence based typing

SE: Shared epitopes

SLC34A1: Solute Carrier Family 34

SSP: Sequence specific primer

T: Thymine

TBE: Tris-Boric acid-EDTA

TCR: T-cell receptor

TFDP2: Transcription Factor Dp-2

TGF-b: Tumor growth factor-b

TNF: Tumor necrosis factor

UNOs: United network for organ sharing

VCAM: Vascular cell adhesion molecule

VXM: Virtual cross-match.

WHO: World health organization

XM: Crossmatch

Chapter-1

Introduction

Chapter-1

Introduction

Despite several decades Kidney transplant is offered as renal replacement therapy to end stage renaldisease (ESRD) patients who suffer morbidity and mortality. Hence, there is a need for developing novel approaches. There seems to be a possibility of developing prognostic or predictive multigene DNA array tools that could help in identifying 'high-risk' ESRD patients and it might lead to personalized treatment strategies for both ESRD and transplantation.

There are two different types of renal failure - acute and chronic. Acute renal failure has an abrupt onset and is potentially reversible. Chronic failure progresses slowly over the period of at least three months and can lead to permanent renal failure. Chronic kidney disease (CDK) affects about 10% of the world's population. Due to the lack of accurate national data collection, the incidence of CKD in India is not clear.

1.1 Incidence -World scenario chronic kidney diseases

End-stage renal disease (ESRD) occurs when the kidneys are no longer able to function at a level that is necessary for day-to-day life. More than 85% of ESRD patients require renal replacement therapy. African Americans have a 4-fold or greater risk of hypertensive and diabetic ESRD compared to European Americans and even more risk in the southeastern USA (Bethesda 2003).

Certain conditions, however, are affecting the kidneys that promote greater incidence in women - for example, urinary tract infections that lead to infection and scarring of the kidneys and autoimmune diseases, Rheumatoid Arthritis, and Systemic Lupus Erythematous. In the United States, the approximate number of ESRD cases stands at slightly higher than four lakh (Grassamann et al., 2005). These figures indicate the tip of the iceberg as the incidence of CKD is expected to be thirty times more than that observed for ESRD (Norfords et al., 2006). In United states cases of ESRD are higherthan approximately four lakh (Grassamann et al., 2005).ESRD incidences are increasing its like iceberg tip it is evident that 1 in 10 adults, i.e. over 500 million people worldwide are affected with CKD (Grassamann et al., 2005, Norfords et al., 2006). Out of ~26 million CDK affected adults in the US, nearly 19 million cases are placed in an early-stage category. Diabetes and hypertensive nephrosclerosis incidences are increasing in numbers of CKD compare to figure in 2008 treatment cost of ESRD in USA was nearly $40 billion (Couser et al., 2007). Among newly diagnosed, about 10% ESRD cases undergo transplantation (Couser et al., 2007). Multiple causes e.g., cardiovascular disease, chronic interstitial nephritis (CIN), Hypertension (HTN) Lupus nephritis, Metabolic diseases, Vascular diseases associated with a cardiovascular condition, diabetic nephropathy (DN) are reported to be responsible for renal failure.

In India, the exact prevalence is unclear as there is no central registry for patients. Various studies estimate that the number of new patients diagnosed with ESRD who are started on dialysis or transplantation is over 100,000 per year. This number grossly underestimates the true burden of kidney disease in our country given the inequality in access to health care between urban and rural populations. The most common causes of kidney disease in India among men and women are diabetes and hypertension (S. Chandra Das, 2017). ESRD has reached epidemic proportions in India (Agrawal et al., 2009). In India CKD incidences areapproximately 800 per million population (pmp), and ESRD is 150-200 pmp. This incidence is reported very lower in the developed world, environmental factors along with socioeconomic condition and genetic background of the population may be accountable for progression of ESRD (Agrawal et al., 2005, 2009). Diabetes and hypertension is responsible for 40–60% CKD cases as per recent ICMR (Indian Council of Medical Research) data, the incidence of diabetes has risen to 7.1%, (varying from 5.8% in Jharkhand to 13.5% in Chandigarh) and in urban population (over the age of 40 years) the prevalence is as high as 28% (Raman R.201, Anjana RM, 2011). Likewise the reported prevalence of hypertension in the adult population today is 17% (14.8% from rural and 21.4% from the urban belt). A similar incidence found by Panesar *et al.* is 17.4% (in the age group of 20–59 years) alsoin slum-resettlement colony of Delhi (Panesar S, 2013,Bhadoria AS, 2014)

Ethnic differences in the incidence of ESRD between different ethnicities within developed Nations has been observed. Diabetes nephropathy commonest cause of CKD among Indians (Rajapurkar et al.2012).Authors have focused on the population from a rural belt of Karnataka. The mean age of population was 39.88 ± 15.87 years with 3.82% prevalence of diabetes and 33.62% of hypertension. In India present study population is younger and even the prevalence of diabetes is low despite that the prevalence of stage 3 CKD is reported to be higher (6.3%). Possibility with changing population the difference between urban and rural areas is getting blurred. Undoubtedly, more Indian data needed to validate these findings. (Peterman, 2015). In Indian population an estimated incidence of ESRD of 100 pmp, approximately 100,000 patients might develop ESRD each year.

1.2 Genetic factors in ESRD

ESRD is a complex disease with significant genetic heterogeneity, gene-gene, and gene-environment interactions. Both immunological and non-immunological factors contribute to end-stage renal Disease.CKD development is linked with family history which is Nine-ten - fold receptive for developing ESRD. The racial variation is also observed towards susceptibility for ESRD among Hispanic American, African American, and resident Americans (Pugh et al., 1996) Populations. Among developing countries, the incidence of ESRD is approximately 9-fold among from American ethnic background (freedman et al., 1993, 1995, 1997, Bergman et al., 1996, Lei et al. 1998). It has been reported that among Caucasians, the first and second-degree relatives are affected more with ESRD as compared to controls (Seaquist et al. 1989). These studies reveal the importance of genetic and environmental factors affecting renal failure. ESRD is prevalent among families having nephropathy associated with type-1 (Freedman 1993) and type-2 (freedman1995) chronic glomerulonephritis (Fredman et al, 1997), diabetes mellitus (Lei et al, 1998) and hypertension (Bergman et al, 1996).

1.3 Biochemical parameters

During ESRD the abnormal biochemical levels have been noticed. ESRD patients showing cardiac arrest (Brenner & Rector's The Kidney, 2012) having potassium (K+) and Magnesium (Mg+2) levels increased with the feeling of weakness. It has been reported that during early renal failure (RF), urea and serum creatinine levels increase in advanced (creatinine greater than 10 mg/dL) RF. Chloride concentration initially increased as a function of creatinine in early RF, but decreased in advanced RF, whereas the anion gap increased throughout RF. Mean serum phosphate concentration also increased steadily but remained below the upper range of normal (4.7 mg/dL) during early RF without the use of phosphate binders. These data suggest that different biochemical parameters change at different rates as a function of the severity of renal dysfunction; although phosphate retention may occur, hyperphosphatemia is not a hallmark of early RF (Hakim RM et.al Am J Kidney Dis. 1988).

ESRD is also known as chronic kidney disease (CKD) or chronic kidney failure (CRF). It is a condition in which kidneys stop functioning putting life is in danger. During the end-stage (1 to 5 stages) kidney disease, the kidneys no longer can remove wastes and concentrate urine, hence electrolyte balance is lost. It usually occurs when chronic kidney failure (CRF) has progressed and kidney function is less than 10% of normal. CRFratiois equal in both male and female patients and is independent of age (Soyibo and Barton 2006).Patients causing the accumulation of waste product in blood like urea and creatinine (>1.5 mg/dL/Lit/hr.) leading to uremic toxicity in which the Glomerular Filtration Rate (GFR) is decreased among those a primary indication for renal replacement therapy either dialysis or kidney transplantation. An individual suffering from renal ailment is declared to be affected with CKD when GFR is less than 60 ml/min/1.73m2 for a more than three months (Inker et al. 2014). Increased proteinuria/albuminuria, abnormal size of kidney and presence of hematuria like conditions are the markers of kidney damage. Patients are classified according to GFR, ranging from stages 1 and 2 which indicate urinary abnormalities with preserved renal function to stage 4 and 5 representing advanced form of CKD and ESRD, usually characterised with a GFR < 15ml/min/1.73m2 (Inker et al. 2014). CKD categorization is performed as per the guidelines prescribed by apex bodies like International Society of Nephrology and the American Kidney Foundation.

1.4 Symptoms of ESRD

ESRD is commonly associated with anorexia, malnutrition, and inflammation (Choi et al 2009, Schwedt et al 2009). The high prevalence of inflammation in ESRD is of high clinical importance as evidenced by high C-reactive proteins (CRP) (Tripepi et al 2005).The causes of the high prevalence of elevated CRP levels remain unknown, although it seems conceivable to speculate that both dialysis-related and non-dialysis related factors, such levels of CRP appear to reflect generation of pro-inflammatory *IL-1, IL-6* cytokines and tumor necrosis factor -α (*TNF-α*), and endothelia and other inflammatory mediators including eicosanoids, complement activation products, platelet-activating factor, chemokines, and lipid-derived chemotactic factors has been demonstrated human glomerulonephritis (Kimmel et al 1999; Sawitzki et al 2009). The circulating leucocytes release cytokines such as *PDGF, TGFb,* and *bFGF* which stimulate extracellular matrix (ECM) production by interstitial cells such as fibroblasts causing interstitial fibrosis. Uremic macrophages exhibit increased HGFIN gene and protein expression and heightened expression of proinflammatory and a suppressed expression of anti-inflammatory cytokinesHematopoietic growth factor inducible neurokinin-1 (HGFIN). ESRD-induced inflammation and vascular and soft tissue calcification expression found in the pathogenesis. (Pahl et al 2009).

Kidneys are very small organ in the body; they perform a very important role of filtration, but sometimes get deranged due to the gradual fall in glomerular filtration rate (GFR) with increasing age (Levi et al 1993). Fortunately, the small decrease in renal function is of no clinical significance. However, the rate of renal function loss is significant in patients with a renal disorder, even if the primary insult or underlying disease activity has already abated. This results in several metabolic disturbances (Riegersperger et al 2007). The rate of loss of renal function is different in different individuals even if they have the same underlying cause (Riegersperger et al 2007) indicating the multifactorial nature of the end-stage renal disease. Increased morbidity and mortality is often associated with a chronic disease condition. The frequency has increased significantly among middle-income nations across the globe in comparison to developed countries (WHO, 2005).

1.5 Kidney transplant

Renal transplantation leads to long term survival for ESRD patients in developed and developing countries. Another option is patients are on regular dialysis which is one of the methods to remove the waste product of the body and maintain the electrolyte Balance. About 5000 to 7000 renal transplants are performed in India each year. Most of the time donors are living related in Indian scenario as cadaver transplantation remains a social problem (Shroff et al 2003). Slowly numbers of the kidney of transplant (KT) are increasing, and approximately 10,000 KT in 2018 at different centers of India. Although, here the majority of donors were living, the number of deceased donors is increasing each year. Looking at the Indian scenario of increasing number of CKD and ESRD patients, it is an alarming situation. There is an acute need to increase transplant rate to meet the demand, there is a severe scarcity of organ/donors. Legally in India only living related donors are permitted to donate an organ. Deceased donor program is not yet regular affair.

1.6 Factors influencing transplant outcome.

Factors influence long term kidney transplant outcome, which is defined by patient death or renal dysfunction leading to graft loss. Factors are the quality of the transplant, living donorskidneyshowing a positive impact, while kidneys from expanded criteria donors show poor outcome. The scores exist to predict mid- to long-term outcomes is clinicopathological and avoid the transplantation of kidneys display inferior results. The major factors for recipient areage, disease recurrence, HLA matching, HLA immunization, ethnic background, time on dialysis, and cardiovascular comorbidities. Renal function based on estimated GFR and/or proteinuria values, is a result of all these factors. Delayed graft function has a harmful long-term impact, as does the level of renal function impairment either in stable condition or in case of progressing dysfunction.Although current immunosuppressive therapy are highly efficient in preventing acute rejection, the burden of specific (diabetes, nephrotoxicity) and nonspecific (infection and cancer) side effects have considerable negative long-term consequences that may well be worsen in the future because of aging process in both donors and recipients. Therefore safer immunosuppression strategies is needed to improve long-term outcomes.

1.7 Immunological factors leading to graft rejection.

Literature shows that 10% to 20% of transplant patients suffer rejection in the first year while 20% to 50% of patients lose their graft within ten years because of chronic Rejection. Along with others, factors of rejection play a major role in long term graft outcome. Our study group patients suffered rejection episodes about 24.9%. Those patients who had good HLA match with donor had fewer rejections and better outcome so after five years survival rate of this group is 89.4%.

The central mechanism of allograft rejection involves T-cell alloreactivity that stimulates an immune response through various cellular interactions. Recipient's T cells recognize foreign MHC antigens by two distinct routes: (I) Direct recognition of allo MHC molecules presented by allogeneic dendritic cells, and (II) Indirect presentation of donor MHC molecules presented by recipient's antigen-presenting cells (APCs). Adhesion molecules like ICAM-*1*, VCAM-1, etc., mediate the T-cell binding to APCs. MHC class-II molecules interact with CD4+ Th cells via three signals: TCR-MHC class-II interaction, B7 (1 and 2) – CD28 or CTLA4 interaction and CD40-CD40L interaction (Schiffl et al 2001), which cause a stimulatory effect on T-cells (Figure 1) The activated T-cells secrete various cytokines that produce a cascade of signals evolving all reactive immune responses. Simultaneously, MHC class I –TCR interaction activates CD8+ Tc cells to secrete cytotoxic attack molecules, granzymes and perforins (Caglar et al 2002; Ross 1999; Schiffl et al 2001). Other important immunological molecules are various growth factors and chemokines and their receptors (Elhage et al 2001; Huber et al 1999; Piggott et al 1992; Yudkin et al 2000).

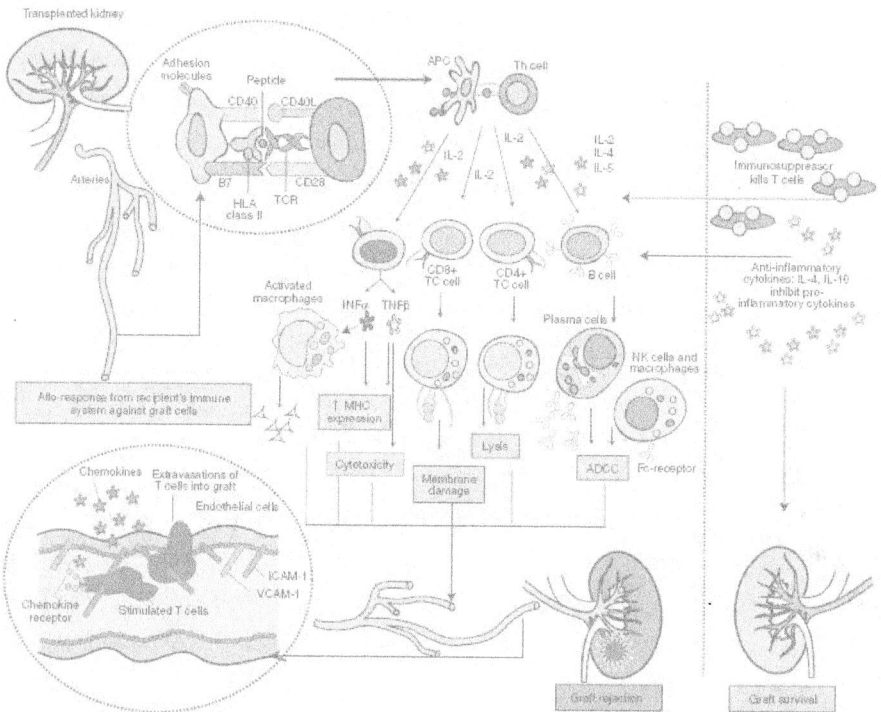

Figure 1.1 Immune mechanisms involved in renal allograft rejection. ADCC = antibody-dependent cell-mediated cytotoxicity; APC = antigen presenting cells; *ICAM-1* = intercellular adhesion molecule 1; *INF*= interferon; *IL*= interleukin; MHC= major histocompatibility complex; NK= natural killer cells; TCR=T-cell receptor; *TNF*= tumor necrosis factor; *VCAM-1*= vascular cell adhesion molecule-1) (Adopted from Khan et al 2006).

To explain the role of different markers, sufficiently detailed studies are required in which genotype, the protein product and the specific phenotype are analyzed in relation to outcome. The recent developments in the field of genetics have opened up entirely new horizon to understand the impact of genotype on disease development and progress and thus offer new options and strategies for treatment (Nordfors et al 2005). It seems to be possible to have a more precise approach for the identification of "high-risk" ESRD patients and the development of accurate individual treatment strategies in the near future. For this purpose, integrative studies on genotype-phenotype associations and impact on clinical outcome are needed.

After renal transplantation, the main complication arises is the rejection. Heavy immunosuppression's are given to patients to avoid rejection episodes.. The major concerns among the transplant biologists, however, is that why there are rejections in spite of the heavy immunosuppression and matching at HLA loci. This may be because of molecular pathways interplaying in the effective immune response that contribute to the heterogeneity of the graft outcome. Therapeutic and prognostic heterogeneity of organ injury is currently impossible to predict. The lack of event and patient therapeutic individualization results in inadequate immunosuppression, resulting in confounding clinical outcomes varying from rejection to malignancy.

1.8 Rejection

Pathogenesis of acute and chronic renal allograft outcomes. The antigenic targets, the mechanisms of T and B cell activation that result in the production of antibody, the complement cascade, methods of antibody detection which are commonly used are complement meditated cytotoxicity, flowcytometry crossmatch and single antigen test by Luminex , and the evidence that alloantibody-mediated mechanisms are active in acute and chronic rejection by graft biopsy.

T cell-mediated inflammation is a central process in allograft rejection. To prevent and treat allograft rejection, immunosuppressive drugs have been directed against T cells. The newer generations of these drugs have improved rates of acute cellular rejection and graft survival; acute rejection does still occur as does the long-term chronic rejection. It was the development of the immunohistochemical process for visualization of complement split product C4d in graft tissue that first provided concrete evidence linking antibody binding and complement activation in renal allografts to the mechanism by which damage occurs in this setting (**Coresh J, 2007**). We now recognize that alloantibodies play a role in rejections that do not respond to T cell therapies and, indeed, require targeted therapies that address various mechanisms by which they exert their effects. Newer and more sensitive technologies for serum antibody screening are allowing for a clearer delineation of the relationship between antibodies and acute/chronic allograft pathologies and their attendant clinical outcomes. The discussion is antigenic targets of the humoral alloimmune response, the mechanism of antibody generation, the pathophysiology of antibody-mediated cell damage, the phenomenon of accommodation, and overview of the current understanding and classification of antibody-mediated syndromes, including the evidence that antibodies are active in these clinical syndromes and presently available therapies.

1.9 Post-transplant Monitoring of organ transplants

In recent years, new methodologies have been developed to monitor various organ transplants. In kidney transplant patients the common method to assess renal function is by measuring serum creatinine levels. Although elevated levels of serum creatinine is suggestive of rejection, cyclosporine-induced nephrotoxicity might also be responsible for the fate of transplant survival. Histopathological examination of a renal biopsy canpermit a differential diagnosis between rejection and cyclosporine toxicity. In immunostaining of renal tubular cells, a main target of infiltrating T cells, shows increased expression of HLA class II antigens during rejection.

Acute rejection episodes are treated with increased immunosuppression mostly in the form of a bolus treatment with steroids or administration of OKT3 or other anti-lymphocyte antibodies or IVIG and plasmapheresis protocol to remove circulating antibody. Early detection of chronic rejection is necessary for effective immunotherapeutic Intervention. Many other factors are also promoting rejections.

In this study we want to understand the roles of various antibodies, and common infections encountered by the recipients during post-transplant period in the outcome of graft survival. To work in line with the objectives of our study, following information was taken into consideration

- HLA typing to study donor-recipient HLA profiles, better match –Better survival.
- Detecting pre and post-transplant formed circulating antibodies and find out relevance.
- Pre and post-renal transplant immune monitoring to guide the requirement of immunosuppression.
- Risk level of MFI (mean fluorescence intensity) of HLA antibodies [DSA].

In the review section, we have discussed in detail the mechanisms of antibody-mediated rejection and the role of CMV, EBV, BKV, HCV, HBsAg infections in renal transplant further we have explained.

Following is the organization of the thesis:

- **Chapter 1:** Deals with the general introduction related to end-stage renal disease and rejections.
- **Chapter 2:** This chapter deals with the review of literature related to rejection under the following headings
- 1 Role of CMV, BK, HBsAg, HCV, and Epstein-Barr viruses (EBV)
- 2 Antibody-mediated rejection.
- 3 Role of donor-specific antibodies.
- **Chapter 3:** This section deals with the detailed methodology of all the techniques like CDC (complement-mediated cytotoxicity), FCXM (flow cytometry cross-match), SA (single antigen), and HLA (human leukocyte antigen) in this monograph.
- **Chapter 4:** This chapter deals with all the results and discussed the results in the light of available literature.
- **Chapter 5:** In the last chapter we have summarized and concluded our findings.

Chapter 2

Review of Literature

Chapter- 2

LITERATURE REVIEW

2.1 Functional anatomy of the normal kidney:

Kidneys are bean-shaped organs found in all vertebrates. Humans have two kidneys, which are located on the left and right retroperitoneal spaces. The main function of the kidney is to extract excess water and waste from the blood and secrete it in the urine, while maintaining an appropriate electrolyte balance (**Figure 2.1**). In adult humans the average kidney is about 10-11 centimeters in size. The kidneys receive blood from the renal arteries and blood exits into the renal veins. Each kidney is attached to a ureter, which carries excreted urine to the bladder.

Figure 2.1 Normal anatomy of the human kidney showing the location in the body and major blood vessels.

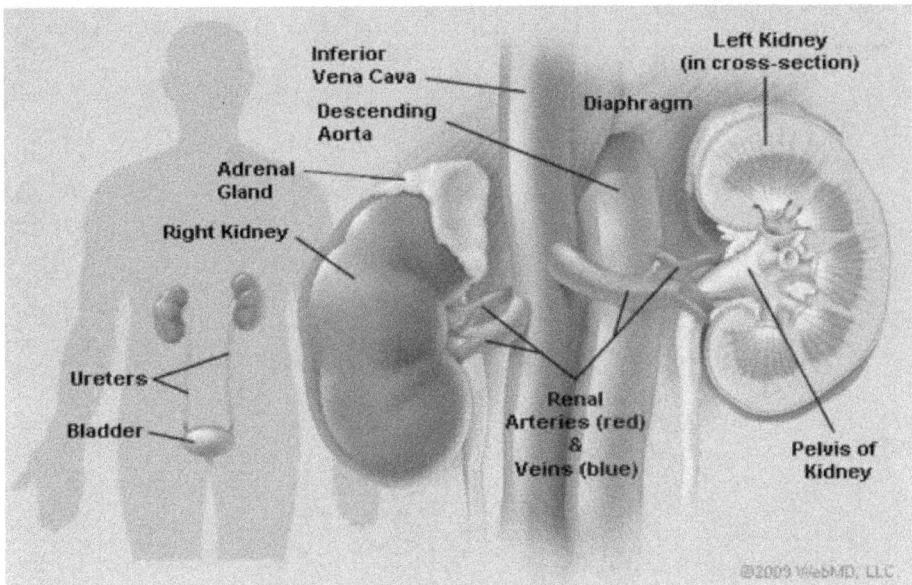

The main structural and functional unit of the kidney is the nephron. Each human adult kidney contains approximately 1 million nephrons. They separate water, ions and small molecules from the blood, filter out waste and toxins for secretion in the urine, and return needed molecules (such as water, sodium, bicarbonate, glucose and amino acids) to the blood. The kidney plays a major role in regulating levels of different minerals such as calcium, sodium, and potassium in the blood. The waste products (including hydrogen, ammonium, potassium, uric acid, and creatinine) are generated from metabolic

11

processes which involve the breakdown of active tissues, ingested foods, and other substances. Filtration is carried out in the glomerulus, which is made up of specialized capillaries within the nephron (**Figure 2.2**). One-fifth of the blood volume that enters in the kidneys is being filtered. The filtered blood goes back into the body and the waste is collected in the form of urine in the kidney's pelvis, where via ureter it enters to the bladder. Kidneys filter about 200 liters of blood and produce about 2 liters of urine daily. In first step of filtration, blood is delivered into the glomeruli by microscopically tiny blood vessels called capillaries. Here, waste products and fluid is filtered from blood, while red blood cells, proteins, and large molecules are retained in the capillaries. In addition to wastes, some useful substances are also filtered out. The filtrate is collected in a sac called Bowman's capsule. The next step in the filtration process is the tubules, which are lined with highly functional cells which process the filtrate, reabsorbing water and chemicals useful to the body while secreting some additional waste products into the tubule.

Figure 2.2 Blood flow in the nephron

The Nephron

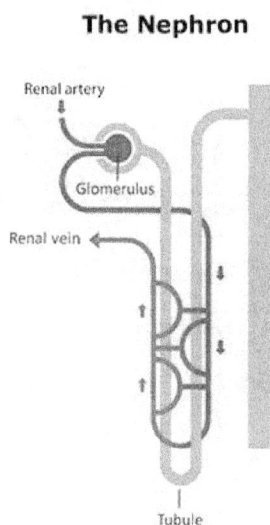

The kidneys also carry out functions independent of the nephron. For example, they convert vitamin D to an active form, called calcitriol, which regulates the absorption of calcium and phosphorus from food promoting bone strength. They are involved in the synthesis of the hormones, erythropoietin that regulates erythropoiesis and rennin, which is involved in the regulation of mineral balance, blood volume, and blood pressure. In addition, the kidney contributes to the degradation of hormones such as insulin and parathyroid hormone.

2.2 Chronic kidney disease: Chronic kidney disease (CKD) includes conditions that damage kidneys and decrease their function (https://www.kidney.org/atoz/content/about-chronic-kidney-disease). With the disparity in kidney function, there is an accumulation of water, waste and toxic products such as creatinine in the blood. Patients with CKD may develop hypertension (which may be a cause or effect of CKD), anemia, mineral and bone disorders, acidosis, cholesterol disorders, and nerve damage. Individuals with kidney disease also have an increased risk of heart and blood vessel disease. These problems may appear gradually over a long term.

2.2.1 Causes of CKD:

The two main causes of CKD worldwide are diabetes and high blood pressure, which are responsible for approximately two-thirds of the cases (https://www.kidney.org/atoz/content/about-chronic-kidney-disease).

Other conditions that affect the kidneys include:

- Glomerulonephritis: A group of diseases that cause inflammation and damage to the kidney's filtering system. These disorders are the third most common type of kidney disease. Glomerulonephritis may be acute or chronic. Acute disease may occur as a result of streptococcal infection.
- Inherited diseases: Polycystic kidney disease causes large cysts to form in the kidneys and damage the surrounding tissue. Other inherited kidney diseases include Alport syndrome (inherited disease of the glomerular basement membrane) and various metabolic diseases.
- Malformations utero: For example, a narrowing may occur that prevents the normal outflow of urine and causes urine to flow back up to the kidney. This causes infections and may damage the kidneys.
- Lupus and other diseases that affect the body's immune system.
- Obstructions caused by problems like kidney stones, tumors or an enlarged prostate gland in men.
- Repeated urinary tract infections.
- Regular use of analgesics such as acetaminophen (Tylenol), ibuprofen (Motrin, Advil), and naproxen (Naprosyn, Aleve) can cause analgesic nephropathy. Certain other medications may damage the kidneys.
- Other factors include HIV infection, sickle cell disease, heroin abuse, amyloidosis, and certain cancers.

2.2.2 Measurements of kidney function:

Blood urea nitrogen (BUN) and serum creatinine may be used to monitor kidney disease. Urea is the waste product of the breakdown of protein, and creatinine is of normal muscle breakdown. The levels of these substances rise in the blood as kidney function worsens. Though, the available tests for kidney function are not very sensitive as normal values appear to vary with factors such as age, race, gender, and body size.

The glomerular filtration rate (GFR) is the primary measure of kidney function, since many of the functions of the kidney are related to the GFR. The classification of chronic kidney disease is also based on the GFR value. The test estimates the amount of plasma passing through the glomeruli each minute. The GFR falls with the progress of kidney disease. The normal GFR is about 100 to 140 mL/min in men and 85 to 115 mL/min in women. It decreases with age. The GFR is calculated from the amount of waste products (e.g., creatinine) in a 24-hour urine or by using markers administered intravenously (e.g. inulin, isotopes). However, conducting these tests are not feasible for measuring GFR in routine clinical practice [Giles PD and Fitzmaurice DA, 2007].An estimated GFR (eGFR) may be calculated by using the results of a serum creatinine, patient age, body size, and gender. The serum creatinine level can be affected by patient diet, pregnancy, obesity, and muscle mass; thus, a blood test for cystatin C may also be used as a confirmatory calculation. However, eGFR values have limitations and may overestimate or underestimate a patient's kidney function. Therefore, multiple methods for measuring and estimating GFR may be recommended [Steubl D and Inker LA, 2018]. Analysis of the urine (urinalysis) is also used for evaluating the function of the kidneys. The presence of more than minimal quantities of albumin in the urine suggests kidney damage. The ratio of albumin and creatinine in the urine provides a fine estimate of albumin excretion per day. In addition, the microscopic examination of the urine to detect red and white blood cells and the presence of casts and crystals (solids) can also be diagnostic (https://www.ncbi.nlm.nih.gov/pmc/articles/PMC4089693). Other blood tests may also be abnormal in the presence of CKD. There may be imbalances in electrolytes, especially potassium, phosphorus, and calcium. The acid-base balance of the blood is also disrupted. Decreased production of the active form of vitamin D can decrease level of calcium in the blood. The failure of diseased kidneys to excrete phosphorus causes its levels in the blood to rise. Testicular or ovarian hormone levels may also be disturbed. Lastly, because kidney disease disrupts blood cell production and shortens the survival of red cells, the red blood cell count and hemoglobin may become low (anemia).Ultrasound may also be used in the diagnosis of kidney disease. In general, kidneys are shrunken, may be normal or even large in size in cases caused by adult polycystic kidney disease, diabetic nephropathy, and amyloidosis. Ultrasound may also be used to diagnose the presence of urinary obstruction, kidney stones and also to assess the blood flow into the kidneys. A biopsy of the kidney tissue may be done in cases in which the cause of the kidney disease is unclear.

2.2.3 Stages of CKD: CKD is commonly divided into five stages of increasing severity based on GFR levels (Giles and Fitzmaurice): provide the details of reference

Stage 1 – Normal GFR (>90 ml/min/1.73m^2) with other evidence of kidney damage.

Stage 2 – Mild decrease in kidney function (GFR 60 to 89 ml/min/1.73m^2) with other evidence of kidney damage.

Stage 3 - Moderate decrease in kidney function (GFR 30-59 ml/min/1.73m^2).

Stage 4 - Severe decrease in kidney function (GFR 15-29 ml/min/1.73m^2).

Stage 5 - Established kidney failure (GFR < 15 ml/min/1.73m^2 or dialysis).

CKD may progress with no symptoms until only very minimal kidney function is left because the kidneys are able to compensate for problems in their function. Therefore, early diagnosis using blood and urine tests is extremely important.

Kidney function may be maintained at early stages of CKD with proper diagnosis and treatment. Dietary changes (including restrictions of protein, salt, fluid, potassium, and phosphorus) may be recommended. In addition, careful management of the disease process that causes the CKD (e.g. diabetes or hypertension) is needed to prevent further damage to the kidneys.

2.3 Management of end-stage kidney disease (ESRD):

If the diagnosis of CKD occurs too late, or the progression cannot be prevented, then renal replacement therapy is required. Renal function can be restored by dialysis or by kidney transplantation.

Dialysis is the process of removing waste products and excess fluid from the body. Two types of dialysis are there: hemodialysis and peritoneal dialysis (www.webmd.com/a-to-z-guides/kidney-dialysis#1). In hemodialysis, the patient's blood is passed through a filter in a dialysis machine. The filter is designed to mimic the function of the kidney nephrons and remove waste and fluid. In peritoneal dialysis, a dialysate fluid is placed in the abdominal cavity, where it absorbs waste from the small blood vessels in the abdomen. The fluid is then drained away.

A vascular access is needed for hemodialysis so that blood can be moved through the dialysis filter at rapid speeds. Vascular access requires either an arteriovenous fistula (where an artery is joined to a vein), an arteriovenous graft (made of artificial material), or a central venous catheter. Two needles are placed in the access site during dialysis. One needle is for collecting blood to run through the dialysis machine and the other is to return the cleansed blood to the body.

For peritoneal dialysis, a catheter is surgically implanted into the abdomen. It is used to transfer dialysate into the abdomen and remove it when the dialysis is complete [Arnoud Peppelenbosch, 2008].

2.4 Kidney Transplantation:

Kidney transplantation involves taking a kidney from a living related donors, living unrelated donors, or people who have died of other causes (deceased donors), and surgically implanting it into the recipient. For most ESKD patients, kidney transplantation is preferred to dialysis. With a transplant the quality of life is improved because dialysis patients undergo treatments multiple times a week for multiple hours at a time. Patients on dialysis may be too sick or lack the energy to allow them to work and lead a normal life. But even more importantly, transplantation confers a huge survival advantage to the patient [Lam AQ, 2019]. Due to the limited of available donors, however, all eligible patients may not receive a transplant. Also, kidney transplantation requires a major surgical procedure with its inherent risks, and patients are required to be on immunosuppressive drugs, which may cause significant side effects.

Transplant patients who receive a live donor kidney have a 5-year survival of 87% and those who receive a kidney from a deceased donor have a 5-year survival of almost 75%. (https://www.emedicinehealth.com/chronic_kidney_disease/article_em.htm#can_chronic_kidney_disease_be_pre vented). Studies that have compared the survival of patients who have been accepted for kidney transplantation and undergone surgery (the transplant group) compared to the survival of those who have not yet received a transplant (waitlist group). Most of these studies have clearly shown that patient survival is better with kidney transplantation than with dialysis [Oniscu GC, 2005; Rabbat CG, 2000]. In one study of the kidney transplant waiting list in the USA, the annual death rate was much lower among transplant patients vs. those still on dialysis (3.8 vs. 6.3 deaths/100 patient-years) [Wolfe RA,1999]. Unfortunately, there are currently not enough donors for all the recipients who could benefit from a kidney transplant.

2.4.1 Factors affecting kidney transplant outcomes:

A person who needs a kidney transplant undergoes a number of tests to determine the characteristics of his or her immune system, including HLA typing and HLA antibody screens. The more identical the donor is in these characteristics, the greater the chance of long-term success of the transplant. Transplant surgery is a major procedure which requires 10 to 15 days in the hospital, so recipients must be healthy enough to survive the operation and immediate post-transplant period. All transplant recipients require lifelong immunosuppressant medications to prevent their bodies from rejecting the transplanted kidney. Immunosuppressant medications require careful monitoring of blood levels because increased the risk of infection as well as some types of cancer.

2.5 HLA system:

Human leukocyte antigens (HLA) are the human version of the major histocompatibility complex (MHC), which plays an integral part in the maintenance of immune surveillance. They are also the main targets during transplant rejection. A donor with an identical HLA system can donate tissue more successfully than the one who is not matched. There are two classes of HLA antigens, based on structure and function. Both class I and II HLA molecules have a similar molecular structure specialized in the presentation of peptides, with a groove to place the peptide being presented to T cells. The floor of this groove is a beta-pleated sheet, and the walls of the groove are alpha helixes. These structures are coded by exon 2 and 3 of class I genes and exon 2 of class II genes. Class I molecules are dimmers with a polymorphic heavy (alpha) chain coded by the HLA-A, HLA-B and HLA-C genes, and a light chain formed by the monomorphic beta-2-microglobulin (**Figure 2.3**). The HLA genes express their gene products on the cell surface. Class I genes have a broad expression and are found on all nucleated cells as well as platelets.

Figure 2.3 Structure of an HLA Class I molecule

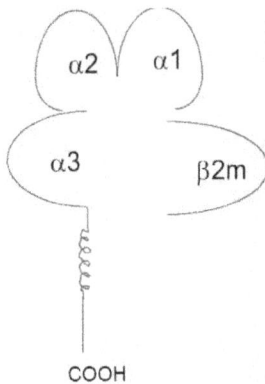

Class II molecules are heterodimers formed by an alpha (heavy) chain coded by the HLA-DRA1, HLA-DQA1 or HLA-DPA1 genes; and a beta (light) chain coded by HLA-DRB1, HLA-DRB3/4/5, HLA-DQB1 or HLA-DPB1 genes (**Figure 2.4**). They have a more restricted expression, and are constitutively expressed on antigen-presenting cells such as dendritic cells, macrophages and B cells. They may also be induced on other cells during inflammation.

Figure 2.4 Structure of an HLA Class II molecule

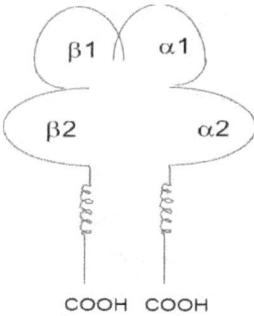

DRB1 and DRB3/4/5 molecules form heterodimers with DRA1, DQB1 with DQA1, and DPB1 with DPA1. All these genes are clustered together on the short end of chromosome 6 in the order shown in figure 5.

Figure 2.5 Genes of the HLA system.

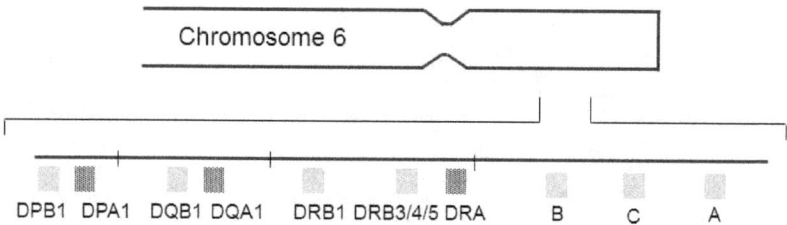

The function of the HLA molecule is to present antigen to T cells. The antigen is bound as a peptide in the antigen-presenting site, or peptide-binding groove, of the molecule which is where most of the sequence polymorphism between different HLA alleles is found. The molecule also includes trans-membrane and cytoplasmic regions. A simplified drawing of the structure of HLA Class I and Class II molecules is shown in (**Figure 2.6**) followed by the exon layout of the genes.

18

Figure 2.6 Antigen recognition sites

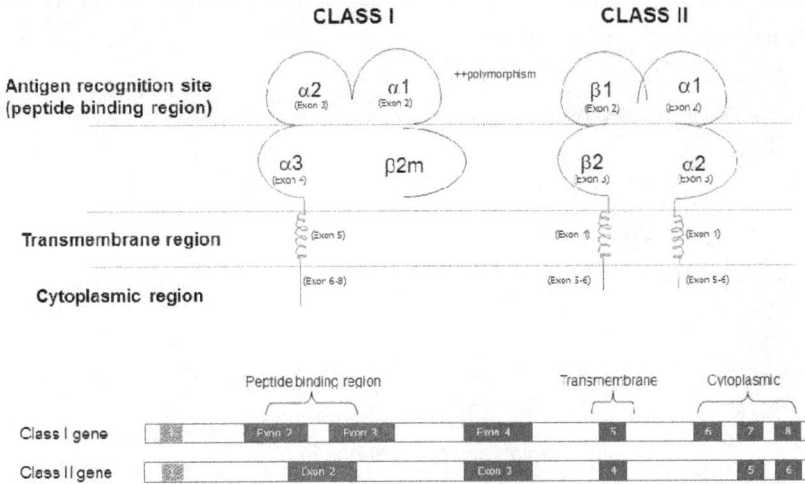

Peptides of intracellular origin are generated in the cytosol by the proteasome and are transported by the TAP transporter into the endoplasmic reticulum, where they bind to HLA class I molecules. Peptides of extracellular origin presented by HLA class II molecules are generated in acidified intracellular vesicles. HLA molecules bind a wide variety of peptides to be presented to T cells. Which peptides can be presented to T cells is determined by the polymorphism of the HLA molecules.

All HLA loci are polymorphic (have more than one allele) and some are extremely polymorphic – for example, HLA-B has over 6000 alleles ["HLA alleles numbers", from hla.alleles.org/nomenclature/stats.html, accessed 26.08.19]. The polymorphism of HLA alleles is mostly the result of gene conversion, that is, the transfer by recombination of a small fragment of DNA from one allele to another allele in the same locus. Only to a much lesser extent is a point-mutation the source of HLA polymorphism. This fact makes the polymorphism of HLA genes very informative, in the sense that sequence variations are not unique to a particular allele but common to many alleles, greatly facilitating the design of PCR primers and hybridization probes.

HLA genes are co-dominantly expressed, so each individual has two HLA antigens from each locus (i.e. two A, two B etc.). The genes are closely linked to each other and are usually inherited as a set, or haplotype, from each parent. Thus a child inherits two haplotypes – one from each parent (**Figure 2.7**). There is a 25% chance of any two siblings matching for both or neither haplotype, and a 50% chance of that siblings will be matched for one haplotype (half-matched). Parents are always matched for one haplotype.

Figure 2.7 HLA type of parents represented as haplotypes (a, b, c, d), showing HLA antigens encoded by the closely linked HLA-A, B and DR genes. Possible haplotype combinations that can be inherited by these parent's offspring are shown below.

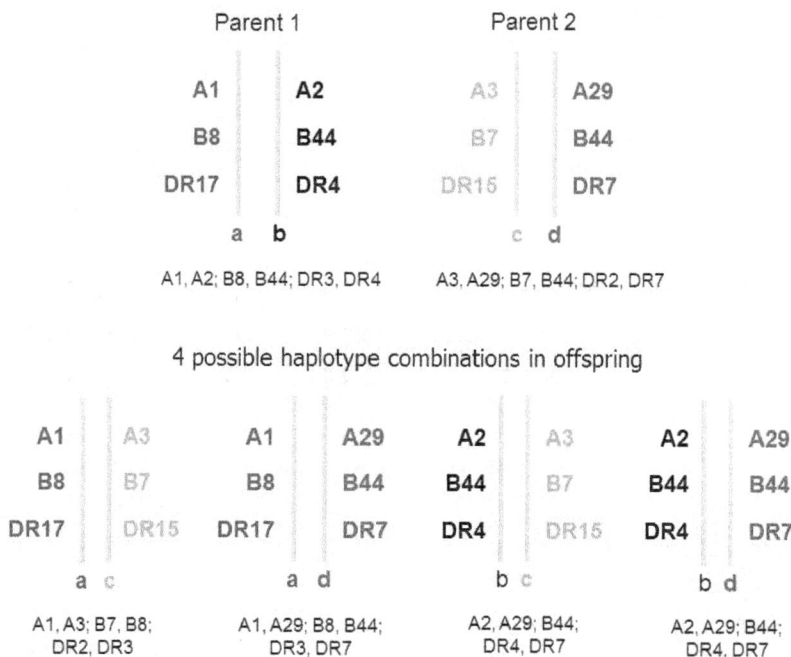

Parent 1		Parent 2	
A1	A2	A3	A29
B8	B44	B7	B44
DR17	DR4	DR15	DR7
a	b	c	d

A1, A2; B8, B44; DR3, DR4   A3, A29; B7, B44; DR2, DR7

4 possible haplotype combinations in offspring

A1	A3	A1	A29	A2	A3	A2	A29
B8	B7	B8	B44	B44	B7	B44	B44
DR17	DR15	DR17	DR7	DR4	DR15	DR4	DR7
a	c	a	d	b	c	b	d

A1, A3; B7, B8;   A1, A29; B8, B44;   A2, A29; B44;   A2, A29; B44;
DR2, DR3   DR3, DR7   DR4, DR7   DR4, DR7

2.5.1 HLA nomenclature:

LA names are assigned by the WHO (World Health Organization) Committee for Factors of the HLA System (hla.alleles.org/nomenclature/committee.html). Historically, antigen names were assigned on the basis of serologic typing methods, where sera were identified that reacted with certain epitopes on HLA molecules. Therefore, the names were assigned for the entire molecule, including both the alpha and beta chain for Class II molecules. Besides recognizing the said antigens, these antibodies were later found to recognize shared or "public" epitopes that were present on a family of related alleles. Antigen names include A, B, C, DR, DQ or DP for the locus name, followed by a number (e.g. A1, A2 etc.). Once DNA typing methods were developed, a new nomenclature system was introduced in 2010 where HLA allele sequences were used to assign names (http://hla.alleles.org/nomenclature). In this system, each HLA allele name has a unique number with up to four sets of digits separated by colons. As shown

20

in **figure 2.8**, the digits before the first colon correspond to the serologic antigen family when possible. The second set of digits refers to the subtypes, with numbers assigned in the order in which the alleles were identified. Allele names with numbers that differ in the second set of digits must differ at one or more nucleotides that change the amino acid sequence of the protein. The third set of digits are for nucleotide changes that do not result in an amino acid change (i.e. non-coding substitutions or silent nucleotide substitutions) and the fourth set of digits are for sequence polymorphisms in the introns or untranslated regions in the genes. The third and fourth sets of digits are included only when necessary, so at a minimum, an HLA allele may include only 2 sets of digits (e.g. A*02:01).

Figure 2.8 Nomenclature of HLA alleles

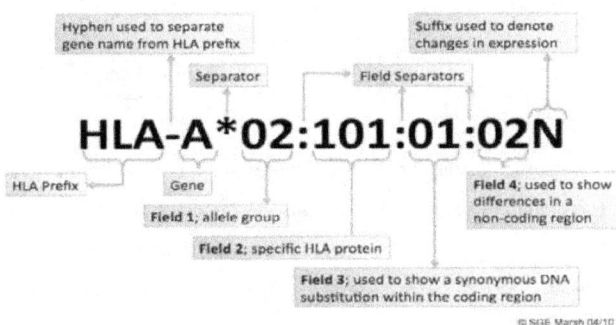

Most solid organ transplant programs now use DNA methods for HLA typing, in which alleles are not usually resolved. Instead, low-resolution typing high-resolution is performed to determine HLA antigens at the level resolvable by alloantibody. In those cases, the serologic format name (i.e. serologic equivalent) may be reported.

Figure 2.9 shows the difference between nomenclatures for HLA antigens vs. alleles. The allele names (top of figure) are given for each gene product. "DQB1*05:01" is an example of a name for an allele encoded by the DQB1 gene. And "DQA1*02:01" is an example of a name for an allele encoded by the DQA1 gene. The products of those two genes (alpha and beta chains) combine to form an HLA molecule called "DQ5" (shown at the bottom of the figure) that is recognized by antibody to DQ5.

Figure 2.9 Naming HLA antigens vs. alleles (note that "HLA" is not shown as part of the names due to space limitations)

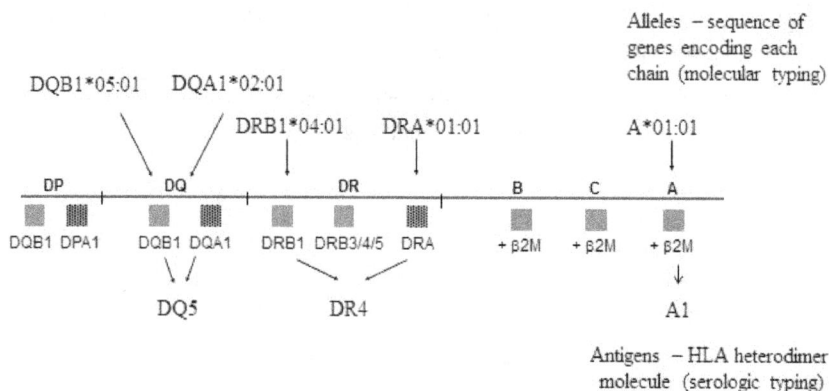

Histocompatibility testing (i.e. testing for HLA antigens and antibodies) is an essential component of a successful kidney transplant program for two reasons [Takemoto et al, 2004]. First, human leukocyte antigens (HLA) play a key role in the cellular and humoral immune responses that determine the outcome of a transplant. Second, the widespread polymorphism of HLA poses a major barrier to successful transplantation. The role of HLA matching in renal transplantation is evolving as advances in immunology increase our understanding of the structure and function of HLA and as improvements in technology have improved our skill to distinguish HLA antigens and the antibodies reactive to them.

HLA antigens be capable of stimulate B cells to produce alloantibodies, which are involved with humoral mechanisms of transplant rejection. Studies have established histopathologic confirmation of humoral rejection with immunostains specific for complement components (especially C4d) and immunoglobulins [Colvin RB, 1996; Feucht HE, 2003]. Although class I antigens controlled by the HLA-A, -B and -C loci are the primary targets of alloantibodies, emerging evidence indicates that antibody reactivity to class II antigens encoded by HLA-DR and HLA-DQ antigens may also result in graft loss [al-Hussein KA, 1994; Schoenemann C, 1998]. Humoral immunity against HLA has also been recognized as a main risk factor for chronic rejection and transplant failure [Terasaki PI, 2003].

2.5.2 HLA matching.

For many years, the practice of HLA matching was based on counting the number of mismatched HLA-A, -B, -DR antigens of the donor. Mismatches result in progressively inferior survival rates [Cecka JM, 1997]. Although HLA matching has been shown to improve outcomes in organ transplantation, a significant proportion of perfectly matched transplants fail, mainly because of non-immunologic reasons having to do with the quality of the kidney or recurrence of the disease. However, others fail because of rejection resulting from allorecognition of donor incompatibilities, which may include molecules not traditionally matched such as minor histocompatibility antigens or MICA [Eric Spierings, 2014].

A poorly matched kidney transplant can do well due to the immunosuppression given to suppress the recipient's immune response to the organ. And if HLA matching were required, it would be far more difficult to identify an appropriate donor and far fewer transplants would be done. In addition, patients often do so poorly on dialysis that receiving a transplant from a poorly matched donor usually results in better patient outcome than waiting on dialysis until a better HLA matched donor could be found [Takemoto et al, 2014]. Bring clarity in this Sentence. Therefore, it is more common for HLA compatibility to be defined in terms of mismatch acceptability mismatches in allo-sensitized transplant candidates that result in a negative cross-match [Claas FHJ, 2009]. This suggests that unacceptable mismatches are antigens react with antibody detectable in the patient sera, where acceptable mismatches are those with no detectable antibody. Transplant centers have the option of maintaining a list of unacceptable mismatches for transplant candidates, which can help expand the search for appropriate donors for broadly sensitized candidates.

2.6 Cross-matching:

The desperate clinical condition of patients and the limitations in the availability of organs dictates the practice of matching recipient antibodies against donor antigens. This has brought the practice of cross-matching to the centre of attention when testing for solid-organ transplants. Although the standard of care is to rely on various forms of cross-matching the patient's serum with donor cells, a more efficient and accurate determination of antibody-antigen matching can be achieve by taking advantage of the new techniques of identification of antibody specificities and DNA-based typing methods. The new techniques of antibody identification using fluorescent beads that each carry a single HLA antigen on their surface allow a more precise characterization of antibody specificities.

The main purpose of HLA typing and lymphocyte cross matching (LCM) in transplantation is to assess donor-recipient immune compatibility and identify the presence of preformed donor-specific cytotoxic alloantibodies in the recipient. It can be tested by serology or molecular techniques.

2.6.1 Increasing the donor pool by kidney paired donation:

One of the main issues limiting organ transplantation worldwide is a lack of donor organs. If a patient with CKD does not have a willing or sufficiently healthy living donor, or they are incompatible with a potential donor due to ABO mismatch or HLA incompatibility, they may then be relegated to many years wait on a deceased donor waitlist, which as noted above is extremely limited in India [Abraham G, 2016].

The concept of kidney paired kidney or donor? (KPD), or kidney exchange, was first proposed by Rapaport in 1986 [Rapaport FT. 1986]. KPD involves pairs in which the donor is incompatible with their intended recipient. In a two-way KPD, two incompatible pairs exchange donor kidneys so that each recipient receives a kidney from the other pair's donor. The classic example is with ABO mismatched pairs, as shown in **Figure 2.10** In this example, both of the donors give kidneys and each of the recipients receives a compatible organ, although from a stranger.

Figure 2.10 Paired Kidney donation

Example of two-way KPD involving ABO mismatched pairs. In this example, donor Mary Smith would like to give a kidney to her husband, Fred Smith, but can't because she is ABO incompatible with him. Donor Emily Jones would like to give a kidney to her sister, Jane Jones, but also can't due to ABO incompatibility. However, Mary can give her kidney to Jane, and Emily can give her kidney to Fred.

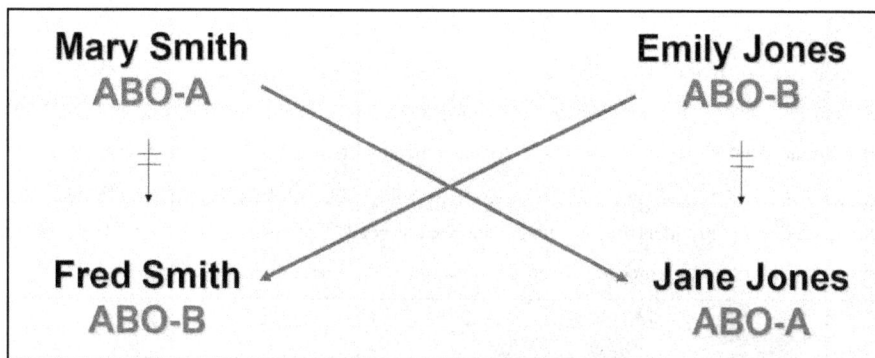

Korea was the first country to establish a formal KPD program [Kwak JY, 1999], but many more countries and programs have introduced KPD since that time. There have also been multiple reports on computerized algorithms for identify optimal exchanges [Roth AE, 2004; Segev DL, 2005].KPD donations can also be done using closed loops of three or more pairs, requiring more sophisticated matching algorithms and software [Ferrari Paulo, 2015]. In the closed loop KPDs, the transplants must be performed simultaneously to ensure that all recipients receive a transplant and to eliminate the risk of any donor withdrawing their Consent. Open "chain" or "domino" KPD may also be done. These chains are often started with a non-directed donor, also known as a "Good Samaritan" or altruistic donor [Matas AJ, 2000]. Such a donor is one who comes forward to donate without having an intended recipient. Adding a non-directed donor into a KPD registry can initiate many more transplants without obligatory matching of a paired recipient. These chains can end with the last paired donor donating to a deceased donor wait-list recipient or acting as a bridge donor, to initiate a future chain [Montgomery Robert A, 2006]. Such chain transplants have greatly increased the number of KPD transplants done in multiple different countries.

Another innovation in the field of KPD is to include compatible pairs in the KPD algorithm, also referred to as "unbalanced" KPD. This altruistic act on the part of the compatible pair may further increase the size of the donor pool and greatly increase the likelihood of finding a compatible donor for difficult to match recipients [Roth Alvin E, 2008]. Although the compatible pair participating in such a program may be disadvantaged due to a delay in transplant that may otherwise have proceeded more quickly, it is also possible to balance that by adding a benefit such as giving them a better HLA matched donor than they would otherwise have received.

One of the first KPD program reports in India was from the IKDRC in Ahmedabad [Kute VB, Vanikar AB, 2014]. There are unique challenges to making KPD successful India, including the fact that non-simultaneous transplants are not allowed, which prevents long KPD chains from being developed. There is also no national waiting list or allocation system, no computerized algorithm, and policies and practices differ between transplant centers. Non-directed anonymous donors are also discouraged. However, the success of the KPD program in Ahmedabad, despite its limitation to mostly 2-way exchanges, demonstrates that a more unified system in India could go a long way to improving access to compatible kidney transplants [Kute VB, 2015].

2.7 Immune response to organ transplants:

The success of renal transplant depends upon both immunological and non-immunological factors. Among immunological factors is allo-recognition through the alloantigens, which include HLA antigens. Alloantigens in the graft tissue are recognized by T cells in different forms. Two pathways of T cell allo-recognition have been implicated in rejection [Moreau et al, 2013]. (A) In the direct pathway, intact allogeneic HLA molecules on the surface of donor tissue are able to directly activate T cells. Donor dendritic cells present in the graft can also directly present alloantigen when they migrate to draining lymphoid tissue shortly after transplantation, where they prime host T cells. The direct pathway results in a very powerful response, as a high frequency of T cells is activated in this manner, and it is thought to trigger early graft rejection. Graft damage is mediated by allospecific effector T cells that infiltrate the graft. Although most professional donor APC will disappear soon after the transplantation, a small proportion may persist in the recipient. It has been suggested that the recognition of donor HLA by alloreactive T cells in the epithelium and the vascular endothelium is an important step in the allograft response. (B).

The second pathway of MHC allo-recognition is referred to as the 'indirect' pathway and involves the internalization, processing, and presentation of alloantigen as peptides bound to recipient MHC molecules. In the indirect pathway, T cells recognize donor allopeptides on self-MHC molecules after being processed and presented by recipient APC. Indirect T-cell alloreactivity can be long lasting because an in situ transplant is a continuous source of donor alloantigens. This mechanism may contribute to the development of chronic rejection [Takemoto paper; 1997].

After renal transplantation the main complications are rejection and infection. To avoid rejection, the patients are kept under a cover of heavy immunosuppression, which may then increase the risk of infection. A literature review of both rejection and infection is in the next section.

2.8 Types of rejection:

Kidney transplants can undergo several types of rejection. The major types are hyper-acute, acute, and chronic rejection. Acute cellular rejection is the most common in allogeneic transplants and in the absence of preformed anti-donor Antibodies. Hyper-acute rejection appears in the first minutes following transplantation and occurs only in vascularized grafts like kidneys. This very fast rejection is characterized by vessels thrombosis leading to graft necrosis. Hyper-acute rejection is caused by the presence of anti-donor antibodies existing in the recipient before transplantation. These antibodies induce both complement activation and stimulation of endothelial cells to secrete Von Willebrand pro-coagulant factor, resulting in platelet adhesion and aggregation. The results of this series of reactions are the generation of intravascular thrombosis leading to lesion formation and ultimately graft loss. Today, this type of rejection is avoided in most cases by checking for ABO compatibility and by excluding the presence of anti-donor human leukocyte antigen (HLA) antibodies by cross-match techniques between donor graft cells and recipient sera.

Acute rejection is caused by an immune response directed against the graft and occurs most often between one week and several months after transplantation, but can occur at any time if immunosuppression is lowered. Acute rejection is diagnosed on histological analysis of a graft biopsy according to an international classification system; the Banff classification for the kidney acute rejection is thought to result from two immunological mechanisms that may act alone or in combination: (1) T-cell-dependent process that corresponds to acute cellular rejection, and (2) B-cell-dependent process that generates acute humoral rejection. With current immunosuppressive treatment, acute rejection occurs in less than 15% of the transplants [Port et al. 2004] in non-sensitized patients.

Chronic rejection, on the other hand, is now the leading cause of graft rejection. Chronic rejection can be mediated by either humoral or cellular mechanisms linked to memory/plasma cells and antibodies. One of the independent risk factors for the development of chronic rejection is the presence of anti-HLA class I and especially class II antibodies [Ozawa et al. 2007]. More than 80% of patients with transplant glomerulopathy have anti-HLA antibodies, 85% being directed against class I or class II antigens [Gloor et al. 2007; Sis et al. 2007; Issa et al. 2008]. Less than half of biopsies (40%) display deposits of C4d suggesting that mechanisms other than complement activation may be associated with CR [Solez et al. 2008].

2.8.1 Antibody-mediated rejection (AMR):

The role of alloantibodies in rejection has been described by many investigators. Halloran's group described a correlation between the prognosis of acute rejection and the production of anti-donor antibodies after transplantation [Halloran et al. 1990]. The presence of antibodies against donor antigens (i.e. donor-specific antibody or DSA) at the time of transplantation was identified as a high risk factor for AMR and patients who develop anti-HLA DSA tend to have inferior long-term graft survival compared to those that do not [Lefaucheur et al. 2008]. It has also been shown that patients who develop de novo DSA after transplantation have an inferior graft outcome [Cooper JE, 2011].

Alloantibodies that develop against the donor organ can recognize several types of antigens [Dragun D. 2008]. Alloantibodies mainly induce AMR by complement-dependent mechanisms. A greater risk of AMR was clearly shown when C4d deposits were associated with DSA [Cosio et al. 2010]. However, in the absence of C4d staining, an association of DSA with altered expression of endothelial genes was also found to be a marker of AMR in kidney patients as the alloantibodies modified the microcirculation [Sis et al. 2009]. NK cells and macrophages are also reported to be involved in AMR in patients with DSA [Moreau et al, 2013]

Several desensitizing protocols have been tested to reduce the DSA that cause AMR, including plasmapheresis or IVIG, as well as treatments targeting complement C5 molecules, proteasome, or $CD20^+$ cells (Raedler et al. 2011; Yoo et al. 2012). A combination of these treatments was shown to improve graft survival outcome [Lefaucheur et al. 2009; Montgomery et al. 2011].

2.9 Immunosuppressive Medications:

Immunosuppressive agents are commonly used in the treatment of autoimmune and immune-mediated diseases and transplantation. Drug development has been rapid over the past decades as mechanisms of the immune response have been better defined [Wiseman Alexander c. 2016]. Commonly used immunosuppressive agents are described here.

2.9.1 Calcineurin Inhibitors (Cyclosporine and Tacrolimus):

The first task of antigen presentation during the allogeneic response is the interaction of the HLA antigen with the T cell receptor. After that, a calcineurin-dependent signaling pathway is induced that results in T cell gene transcription necessary for additional activation. Cyclosporine and Tacrolimus are two commonly used calcineurin inhibitors that inhibit the ability of calcineurin to dephosphorylate nuclear factor (NF) of activated T cells (NFAT), required for translocation from cytoplasm to nucleus, and prevent calcineurin-dependent gene transcription.

2.9.2 Costimulation Blockade by CD80/86:CD28 Targeting (Belatacept):

The co-stimulation interaction of CD80/86 on the antigen- presenting cell with CD28 on the T cell is required for optimal T cell activation. After up-regulation and the generation of an immune response, the T cell expresses CTLA4, which competitively binds to CD80/86 and down regulates the T cell response. To mimic this down regulatory effect, human IgG heavy chains linked with CTLA4 creating a fusion protein, called Belatacept is used to further down regulate the T cell response after organ transplantation.

2.9.3 B cell and plasma cell-directed therapy:

The goals of B cell inhibition include inhibiting not only the humoral response to antigen but also the antigen-presenting cell function and B/T cell interactions that promotes efficient T cell activation and Proliferation. Rituximab is a monoclonal antibody that targets CD20 which is a protein present on pre-B and mature B lymphocytes. The drug leads to B cell depletion through a number of mechanisms, including complement-dependent cytotoxicity, growth arrest, and apoptosis. This results in suppressed

B cell counts for 6–9 months. There is limited data to support its use in AMR, but it is still commonly used. Bortezomib is a drug that inhibits the proteasome that regulates the degradation of proteins in plasma cells. This inhibition leads to inhibition of cell cycling and induction of apoptosis. There is limited data to support the efficacy of this drug in AMR, but it is still commonly used.

2.9.4 Complement Inhibition (Eculizumab):

Eculizumab is a humanized mAb to C5 that inhibits its cleavage to C5a and C5b. Because C5a is a neutrophil chemoattractant and C5b is required to form the C5b-9 membrane attack complex, inhibition of this enzymatic step results in blockade of proinflammatory, prothrombotic, and lytic functions of complement. This drug may be used to treat AMR, although it is very expensive.

2.9.5 Cytokine Inhibition (corticosteroids and Basiliximab):

Cytokines are proteins that are secreted by a variety of cell types and function to direct the initiation, differentiation, and regulation of the immune responses. Pharmacologic targeting of specific cytokines is expected to redirect or inhibit untoward immune response.

Corticosteroids bind to the intracellular glucocorticoid receptor and modulate a multitude of cellular functions by binding to glucocorticoid-responsive elements in the nucleus. Effects on the immune system are also numerous but most clearly related to inhibition of all cytokine transcription by blocking transcription factors. Basiliximab and daclizumab humanized monoclonal antibodies are IL-2 receptor antagonists. Activated T cells produce IL-2, which binds to the IL-2 receptor and induces intracellular signaling to promote the proliferation of T cells. The IL-2 receptor antagonists limit the proliferation of activated T cells.

2.9.6 Intravenous Immunoglobulin:

Intravenous Ig (IVIG) is an Ig pool from several thousand plasma donors to create a product that is IgG rich. IVIG was initially used to provide passive immunity in patients with immune deficiencies (doses of 500 mg/kg monthly). However, research suggests a very diverse immunomodulatory and anti-inflammatory role of IVIG therapy when given in high-doses (1–2 g/kg) [Gelfand EW, 2015]. The mechanisms underlying these effects are broad and not always clear. In kidney transplantation, it has been used for desensitization (inhibition and elimination of preformed HLA or blood group (ABO) antibodies to achieve a negative cross-match and permit transplant) and treatment of antibody-mediated rejection [Jordan SC, 2011].

2.9.7 Polyclonal Antithymocyte Globulin:

Therapeutic antibodies to human lymphocyte antigens have been created by immunizing rabbits with human thymocytes (Thymoglobulin), immunizing horses with human thymocytes (Atgam), or immunizing rabbits with lymphocytes from a Jurkat T cell leukemia line (Fresenius anti-thymocyte globulin [ATG]). Thymoglobulin is most commonly used as an induction agent in kidney transplantation, and/or to treat cellular rejection.

2.9.8 Lymphocyte Depleting Agent (Alemtuzumab):

Anti-CD52 (Campath 1H and alemtuzumab) is a humanized mAb that binds to CD52, an antigen of unclear physiologic significance that is present on both B and T cells. Ligation of CD52 results in depletion of both lymphoid cell lines and can induce lymphopenia within 6-12 months.

2.9.9 Antimetabolites (mycophenolate):

Mycophenolate is an inhibitor of IMPDH, the rate-limiting enzyme of guanine nucleotide synthesis critical for de novo purine synthesis and thus, DNA synthesis. Both T and B lymphocytes are dependent on this pathway for DNA synthesis.

2.10 Infection in renal transplantation.

Infections are a major cause of morbidity and mortality in kidney transplant recipients [Karuthu Shamila and Emily A Blumberg, 2012]. With pre-transplant screening of donor and recipient, vaccination, and post-transplant surveillance and prophylaxis, the impact of infections may be reduced. However, with the introduction of more potent immunosuppression regimens and higher- risk patients, viral infections after renal transplantation have emerged as an important cause of allograft loss. Since transplant recipients may not manifest typical signs and symptoms of infection, diagnosis may be difficult. In addition, treatment regimens may be complicated by drug interactions and the need to maintain immunosuppression to avoid allograft rejection.

One study conducted in the USA reported that the rate of first infections in the first 3 years after kidney transplantation is 45.0 per 100 patient-years [Snyder JJ, 2009]. In India, the rate is likely much higher although studies are not available to confirm that. But the risk factors prevalent in India include tropical climate, poor hygiene and socioeconomic status, high rates of endemic infections, late presentation, and suboptimal diagnostic techniques [Kumar Arun et al. 2016]. The most common causes of post-transplant infection are described in the following sections.

2.10.1 Cytomegalovirus (CMV):

CMV is a genus of viruses in the herpes family that infects people of all ages. Most healthy people have no symptoms when infected, but it can result in serious disease in immunosuppressed individuals such as transplant recipients. CMV infection is the most important viral infection that can occur following kidney transplantation. Direct effects include CMV syndrome (e.g., fever, fatigue, myalgia, and leucopenia) or tissue-invasive CMV diseases (e.g., pneumonitis, gastritis, duodenitis, or colitis). Indirect effects, include acute or chronic graft injuries, allograft rejection, poor graft and patient survival, and acquisition of other infections [Vanichanan Jakapat et al., 2018]. CMV disease has also been found to be an independent risk factor for acute allograft rejection [Reischig T, 2006].

Risk factors for CMV infection include low lymphocyte count, hypogammaglobinemia, donor–recipient CMV serology mismatch, and the use of lymphocyte-depleting agents such as thymoglobulin for treatment. Donor and recipient serology profiles are extremely important in predicting the likelihood of CMV disease. The incidence can reach up to 60% when the donor is positive for CMV IgG and the recipient is negative for it prior to transplant. This is referred to as "D+/R-". The incidence of CMV infection occurs in5% to 30% patients showing positive for CMV IgG R+ [De Keyzer K, 2011], but the incidence can be as high as 50% in patients who received T-cell depletion therapy. Prophylactic treatment with anti-viral drugs (e.g. ganciclovir) is recommended for patients who are at high risk of the disease [Strippoli GFM, 2006].Any time a kidney transplant recipient has any signs or symptoms that may be due to CMV disease, diagnostic testing should be done. Usually, this is done by testing for CMV viremia, which is done by the CMV antigenemia assay or by nucleic acid testing (NAT). NAT is more sensitive [Karuthu and Blumberg 2012].

2.10.2 BK polyomavirus (BKV):

BKV is a nonenveloped, double-stranded DNA virus and a member of the *Polyomaviridae* family. BKV infection after transplantation can cause hemorrhagic cystitis, tubulointerstitial nephritis, ureteric stricture, BKV-associated nephropathy (BKVAN), and premature graft failure. After infection via the oral or respiratory tract, the BKV remains latent in renal tubular epithelial cells and may be reactivated after transplant [Hirsch HH, 2013]. The risk factors for BKVAN include HLA-mismatch, mismatched BKV-specific antibody in the donor and recipient (D+/R−), older age of the recipient, retention of the ureteric stent, reception of anti-rejection treatment, tacrolimus–mycophenolic use, or re-transplantation after graft loss due to BKVAN [Hirsch HH and Randhawa P, 2013]. Often BKVAN occurs in recipients after 3-6 months post-transplantation.

Testing for BKV is done by quantitative DNA virus testing of the urine or plasma. Routine urine screening may be done. However, BK viremia is sensitive for detecting active BKV infection but not specific for nephropathy and has a positive predictive value of only 29% to 67%. Detection of BKV DNA in plasma may represent a better indicator for nephropathy. The gold standard for diagnosing BKVAN is kidney histology, including tubulointerstitial nephritis with cytopathic changes and positive immunohistochemistry using antibodies generally targeting cross-reacting SV40 large T-antigen or BKV antigens, or *in-situ* hybridization for BKV nucleic acids [Fishman JA. 2017].

The mainstay of treatment for BKVAN is to reduce immunosuppressive drugs. The efficacy of antiviral therapy as an adjuvant therapy to immunosuppression reduction is still controversial. However, the reduction of immunosuppressive drugs puts the patient at risk for rejection.

2.10.3 Hepatitis B virus:

Hepatitis B virus (HBV) is a DNA virus from the family *Hepadnaviridae* that primarily targets human hepatocytes, resulting in hepatitis. HBV can be transmitted sexually, mother-to-child, as well as via blood transfusion and organ transplantation [Karuthu and Blumberg 2012]. After infection, the virion DNA is harbored in the nucleus of the hepatocyte, which can cause chronic infection and long-term complications such as cirrhosis or hepatocellular carcinoma. Reactivation of HBV after transplantation is an important concern and is found in up to 94% out of 5% HBsAg positive recipients and antibody to hepatitis B core antigen (anti-HBc), respectively [Degos F, 1988]. Therefore, appropriate pre-transplant evaluation and vaccination for HBV infection is crucial.

2.10.4 Hepatitis C virus:

Hepatitis C virus (HCV) is an RNA virus from the Flaviviridae family. Similar to HBV, HCV can be transmitted via organ transplantation, blood exposure, sexual intercourse, and more uncommonly, through the transplacental. The seroprevalence of HCV in dialysis patients in India has been reported to be approximately 30% [Somsundaram Nirmaladevi and R. Vidhya Rani, 2017]. HCV-positive recipients who undergo kidney transplantation have better survival rates than do patients on the waiting list, but they have a lower rate of graft survival compared to HCV-negative transplant recipients [Morales JM, 2015].

2.10.5 Epstein–Barr virus:

Epstein–Barr virus (EBV) is a gamma herpesvirus with a seroprevalence of more than 90% in adults [Le Jade, 2017]. EBV infection in transplant recipients may range from no symptoms to a variety of

32

illnesses, the most serious of which is a post-transplant lymphoproliferative disorder (PTLD). Kidney transplantation has the lowest incidence of PTLD compared to other types of transplants [Dierickx D, 2018].

2.11 Viral Infection and rejection in Kidney transplant:

Rejection of kidney allograft is frequently associated with a viral infection. A very early study in 1972, prior to the common use of prophylaxis and modern immunosuppression, showed that 72% of CMV-infected recipients developed rejection episodes, while only 17% of the recipients without the virus infection experienced rejection [Lopez C, 1974]. Possible mechanisms of CMV induced rejection have been reported [Borchers AT,1999] and include (1) activation of HLA class I antigen-specific T-cells from cross-reactivity with CMV antigen, (2) direct damage to endothelial cells, and (3) release of pro-inflammatory cytokines e.g., (i.e., IL-1, IL-6, IL-8, and TNF-α. All these may result in an increase in the expression of HLA class II molecules on the allograft and adhesion molecules on the leukocytes and endothelial cells.

In addition, physicians usually decrease immunosuppressive drugs in an infection, which may result in a rejection episode. And then during therapy to treat the rejection, the patient becomes more immunosuppressed, which may promote reactivation of the latent virus. Post-transplant malignancy has also been associated with many viral infections. Disturbing the immune system could lead to either allograft rejection or malignancy. Both types of complications are clearly associated with short graft and patient survival. Certain viral infections are associated with the rejection of the graft or cause malignancy. Transplant physicians must keep the patient's immune system in balance: too much immunosuppression could increase the risk of infection and malignancy, whereas too little immunosuppression could lead to rejection of the graft [Cippà PE, 2015].

2.12 Urinary Tract Infections:

Urinary tract infections (UTIs) are the foremost common bacterial infections, followed by other bacterial infection and septicemia requiring hospitalization of kidney transplant recipients. Alternative added risk factors is deceased-donor transplant, kidney-pancreas transplantation with bladder drainage, prolonged catheterization, uretero-vesical stents, and increased immunosuppressed state; among the transplant recipients women are at greater risk [LorenzE C and CosioFG. 2010]. A retrospective cohort study of 28,942 primary renal transplant recipients from the U.S. Renal Data System database revealed a cumulative UTI incidence of 17% during the first 6 months after transplantation; at 3 years the incidence was 60% for women and 47% for men.

Chapter 3

Materials and Methods

This study discussed 370 ESRD patients that underwent kidney transplant [after permitted by Internal Review Board(IRB) committee of IKDRC]and were followed for five years (infection, rejection and graft survival). Asians specifically of Indian origin(male and female) were enrolled in the study, at the Institute of Kidney Disease and Research Center, Ahmadabad, Gujarat, India. All ESRD patients have two options either they can opt for maintenance dialysis or if they have family-related donor they can opt for living related donor kidney transplant. Voluntary kidney donor from family was identified and screened for general health and fitness, which was obtained from nephrologists, anesthetist, and urologist, and in case of female donor, also, from Gynecologist. Once the patient and donor received fitness clearance they were referred to immunology laboratory for HLA typing and cross-matching.

3.1 HLA typing methods:

The test was originally performed by serotyping, which is the use of specific antibodies to distinguish specific antigens. This test needs lymphocyte preparations from blood; their white blood cells contain the HLA antigen, and specific antibodies to recognize these antigens. Although, due to the unavailability of specific antibodies and differences in the exactness of test results amongst various laboratories, other methods of HLA typing were developed. The serotype-based technique of HLA typing has been substituted by DNA-based study. DNA-based examination detects the sequence of genes that code for the HLA antigens. With the introduction of polymerase chain reaction (PCR), a new means was available for HLA typing.

· Donor and recipient HLA typing performed by molecular methods according to their respective manufacturer's directions.

All recipients and living donors were HLA typed by a sequence-specific oligonucleotide probe (Lab type SSO, One Lambda) and antigen detected by hybridization data analyzed by Fusion software (One Lambda) Or Sequence-specific primers (HLA-A/B/Cw/DR/DQ-SSP) (BAG Healthcare-Germany), after that antigen detection by 2% agarose / ethidium bromide gel electrophoresis, and data analyzed by software (Score software).

3.1.1 Automated DNA purification on the QIAcube

Blood sample collected in EDTA 4ml BD collection tube (purple top)Purification of DNA fromblood using the QIAamp kit, 200 μl buffy coat of whole human blood was used,

3.1.1a Preparation of reagents

When using the QIAamp DNA Blood Mini Kit (50), pipette 1.2 ml protease solvent* into the vial containing lyophilized QIAGEN Protease(store at 2–8°C), as indicated on the label, using the QIAamp DNA Blood Mini Kit (250), To dissolve lyophilized protease added 5.5 ml protease solvent into the vial contain lyophilized QIAGEN Protease. Dissolved QIAGEN Protease is stable for 12 months when stored at 2–8°C. . Buffer AL† (stored at room temperature, 15–25°C) was mixed thoroughly before use. Buffer AL was stable for 1 year. Stored at room temperature. AW1†Buffer (stored at RT, 15–25°C) was supplied as a concentrated, was diluted adding the appropriate amount of ethanol (96–100%) as indicated on the bottle and stable for 1 year. Concentrated buffer AW2* (store at room temperature, 15–25°C) diluted with indicated amount of Ethanol (96–100%). AW2 was stable for 1 year when stored at room temperature.

3.1.1b Preparation of Buffy coat

Buffy coat is a leukocyte-enriched fraction of whole blood. Preparing a Buffy-coat fraction from whole blood is simple and yields roughly 5–10 times extra DNA than an equivalent amount of whole blood. We prepared buffy coat by centrifuging whole blood for 10 minutes at 2500 x g at RT (15–25°C). After centrifugation, 3 different fractions were distinguishable: first upper clear layer is plasma; the second intermediate layer is a buffy coat, containing leukocytes; and the bottom one layer contains concentrated erythrocytes.

Owing to the sensitivity of nucleic acid amplification technologies, the following precautions are necessary while handling QIAamp Mini columns to avoid cross-contamination among sample preparations. Pipette sample into the QIAamp Mini column and avoid wetting the rim of the column. Pipette tips need to be changed for all liquid transfers. The use of aerosol-barrier pipette tips is suggested. Do not touch the QIAamp membrane with the pipette tip. After that centrifuge 1.5 ml micro-centrifuge tubes to remove drops of the lid. QIAamp Mini columns are centrifuged at 6000-x g (8000 rpm) to lower noise. Each solution is transferred through the QIAamp membrane. Extraction of DNA from buffy coat or lymphocytes, high-speed centrifugation is suggested to avoid clogging. All centrifugation must be carried out at room temperature (15–25°C).

DNA quality check and quantification was performed on a spectrophotometer. Good quality of DNA was used for HLA typing test. HLA antigens (A, B, C, DR and DQ) Specific primers (low resolution) were used in pre-doted PCR plate. Total 124 HLA antigens were tested.

HLA typing Test

- DNA primers: short single-stranded DNA to attach the nucleotide sequences that promote synthesis which matches strand of nucleotides
- DNA polymerase: The DNA has a primer bound an enzyme it, goes down the DNA segment assigning DNA building blocks to form complementary base pairs and so synthesizes a complementary nucleotide strand of DNA
- Excess of DNA building blocks called nucleotides (Adenine, Thymidine, Cytosine, and Guanine, abbreviated as: A, T, C, and G, respectively) are there in the solution. These blocks are linked together, they form a nucleotide sequence or a single strand of DNA. After that, these building blocks bind their corresponding building block by hydrogen bonds (A will bond with T and G only with C) a complementary DNA nucleotide sequence is created and bound to the unique single-stranded DNA. After the binding is finished, a complementary double-stranded DNA is created in a specific sequence. This cycle is repeated about 40 times in a thermal cycler machine that mechanically repeats the heating-cooling cycles, the quantity of each DNA sequence doubling every stage the heating-cooling cycle is completed. That primarily was a single small segment of DNA be able to be amplified to about 100 billion copies after 40 copying cycles.

Figure-3.1 Sequence-specific primer (SSP) completely matched primers were used a large number of primer pairs to identify specific sequences results in presence or absence of PCR product

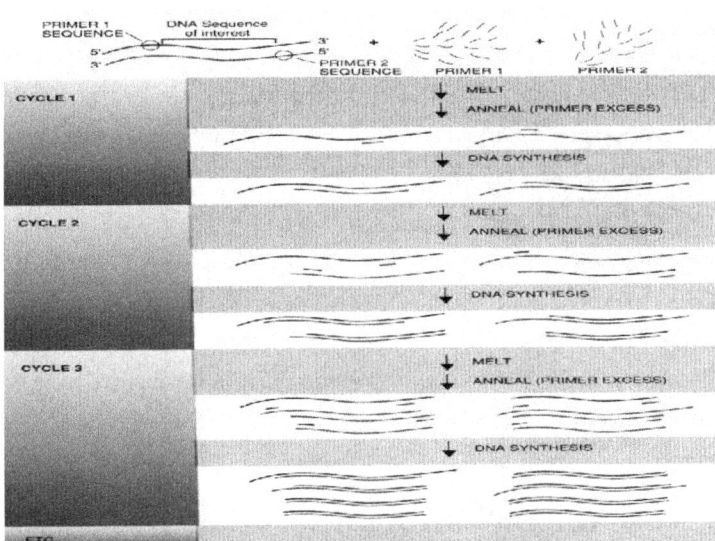

The first is the denaturation step in a PCR cycle. Hydrogen bonds holding the complementary strands of DNA collectively are broken. This second step in a PCR cycle is the annealing step. In the annealing step, the primers anneal, or attach, to the DNA template. After amplification end product was analyzed by Gel-electrophoresis identifying test bands noted positive and analyzed by software. SSP or SSO method positive test (antigens) identified with the help of software by machine-like Luminex.

3.1.2 Amplification –SSP (Sequence-specific primer)

All pre-aliquoted and dried reaction mixtures already include HLA allele and control-specific primers and nucleotides. Amplification optimized to a total volume of 10 μl. required per test of HISTO TYPE HLA-SSP plates. Master-Mix consisting of 10 x PCR-buffer, DNA concentration of 25 – 50 ng per mix, Taq-Polymerase (5 U/μl) and RNA-DNA free distilled water was mixed to make Master-Mix depending on the number of reaction mixes. (E.g. for 24 mixes: 14 μl DNA solution (100 ng/μl) and 236 μl RNA-DNA free distilled water.). After vortexing add 10 μl of this mixture to the pre-dropped and dried reaction mixtures. Tip was changed each pipetting step. Test plate was tightly closed with foil. To dissolve the pellet at the bottom of the plate was shaken and mixed well followed by centrifugation at 2000 RPM for three minutes. All PCR solution should settle on the bottom. Place test plate in the thermal cycler and tighten the lid. Start the PCR program. For Amplification Validated Cycler was used. while using thermal cyclers with a very fast heating and cooling rate, it is recommended to use a reduced ramp rate (~ 3.5°C/sec), because cyclers of different manufacturers perform differently and even each machine of one type may be calibrated differently, it is necessary to optimize the amplification parameters.

3.1.3 Gel electrophoresis

Separation of the amplification products is documented by electrophoresis via a (horizontal) agarose gel. We used electrophoresis buffer, 0.5 x TBE (45 mg. of tris, 45 mg. of boric acid, 10ml of 0.5 mM of EDTA in 500 ml RNA-DNA free deionized distilled water). The gel concentration was 2 % of agarose. Allowed the gel to polymerize at 30 minutes before sample loading. After amplification, test samples were taken out of the thermal cycler and load the total reaction mixtures in each slot of the gel. After that, 10 μl of the DNA length standard was applied for size comparison. Electrophoretic separation was done at 10 - 12 V/cm (with

20 cm distance between the electrodes approx. 200 - 240 V), for 20 min.EtBr (0.5 µg/ml) added to the electrophoresis buffer or the agarose gel. If necessary, excess of EtBr can be removed by soaking the gel in H2O or 0.5 x TBE buffer for 20 - 30 mins. For documentation the PCR amplification visualized using a UV trans-illuminator (220 - 310 nm) and photograph it with a camera and saved image for interpretation. The bands that have the correct size associated with the DNA length standard should be considered positive. All lanes without allele-specific amplification, the 1070 base pair (bp) internal control must be visible. In most cases with an allele-specific amplification, the internal control is weaker or disappears completely. No observable band in the contamination control. If there is a contamination with genomic DNA there will be a band at 282 bp. For the evaluation of bands, HISTO MATCH (Care,) or SCORE (full version) software was used.

Figure 3.2 sequence-specific primers (HLA-A/B/Cw/DR/DQ-SSP) (BAG Healthcare-Germany), followed by 2% agarose/ethidium bromide gel electrophoresis.

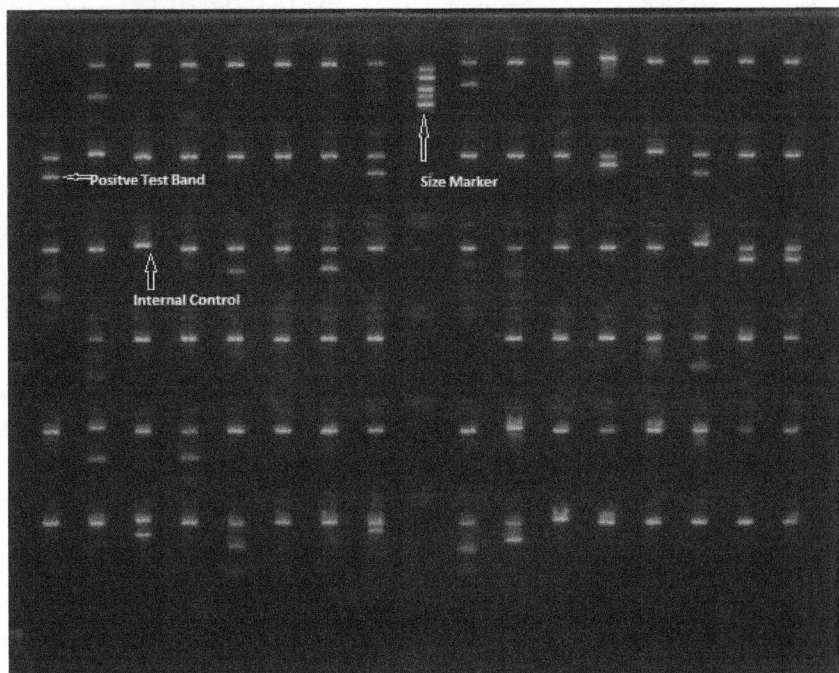

Presence or absence of PCR products is distinguished with Ethidium bromide staining under UV light after agarose gel electrophoresis.

Positive control primers to amplify conserved regions of DNA are incorporated in each amplification.

3.1.4 Amplification –SSO (Sequence specific oligonucleotide)

The concentration of genomic DNA was adjusted to 20ng/µl for that DNA/RNA free water was used. Thermal cycler was warmed up heated lid. The DNA, Amplification Primers and D-Mix, was kept on ice until use. Aliquoted 2 µl genomic DNA to respective wells in PCR tray. Added 18 µl of mixture - of Primer mix (4 µl), D-Mix (13.8 µl), and Taq polymerase (0.2 µl). Cap or seal the PCR tray. Tray was placed in a PCR oven using the LABType SSO PCR program. Amplified DNA was checked on 2.5 % agarose gel (use 5 µl per well).

3.1.5 Denaturation / Neutralization:

In 96 well PCR tray, 5 µl of amplified DNA per well was aliquoted followed byadditionof 2.5 µl of Denaturation buffer per well. Was mixed thoroughly until the mixture changes to a bright pink color. Incubated at room temperature (20° to 25°c) for 10 minutes. Then addition of 5µl per well of Neutralization Buffer. Mixed thoroughly until the mixture turns clear or pale yellow. The tray was placed carefully on the ice.

3.1.6 Hybridization / Washing

Prepare Hybridization mixture by thoroughly mixed 34 µl of Hybridization Buffer and 4 µl of Bead mixture. By adding 38 µl of this Hybridization mixture into respective neutralized DNA. The tray was incubated at 60°c thermal cycler (used PCR Pad) for 15 minutes. Followed by addition of 100 µl of Wash Buffer to each well. Test plate was sealed and spin at 1000 g for 5 minutes. Supernatant was removed. Repeated two more washes for a total of 3 washes.

3.1.7 Labeling: 1X SAPE was prepared by mixing 49.5 µl of SAPE Buffer with 0.5 µl of SAPE Stock. After removal of supernatant from the third wash, 50 µl of 1X SAPE per well was added. Tray was sealed and vortexed thoroughly at low speed. Incubated at 60°c in thermal cycler for 5 minutes. Followed by addition of 100 µl Wash Buffer to each well. The tray was sealed and spin at 1000 g for 5 minutes. Supernatant was removed. Wash Buffer was added to make up the final volume to 80µl. Mixed by pipetting and all samples were transferred to 96 well micro plates for Data acquisition on Luminex XY Platform. The mean fluorescence intensity (MFI) generated by Luminex Data Collector Software. HLA alleles were determined of the samples by matching the pattern of positive and negative bead IDs with the information using HLA Fusion Software.

Figure-3.3 Sequence-specific oligonucleotide probes (Lab type SSO, One Lambda) with positive hybridization detected by Luminex.

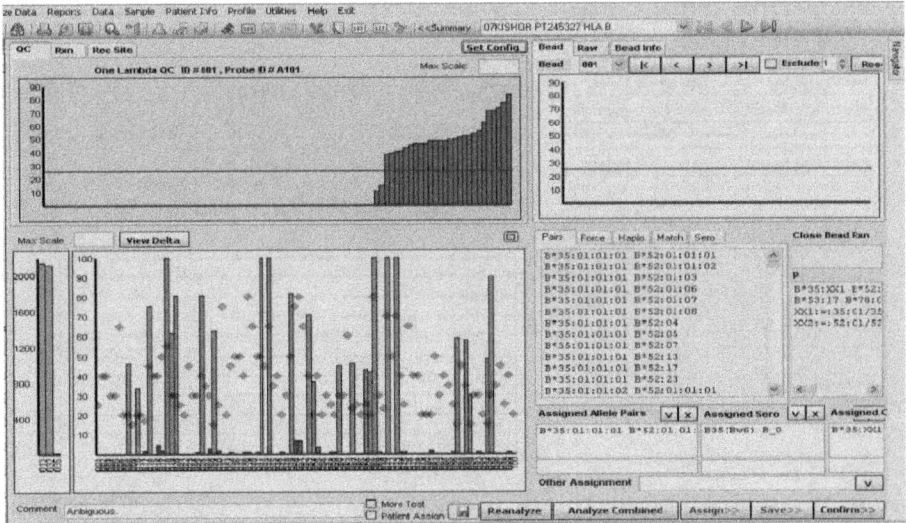

Analysis of SSOP HLA typing by Luminex platform

3.2 Antibody Detection Assays

3.2.1 Lymphocyte cross matching

The pre-transplant cross-match which involves testing the recipient's serum for cytotoxicity against the donor cells (lymphocytes), method was introduced into the testing procedure in the 1960s in the early days of renal transplantation (Terasaki PI1964) The patient's serum and donor cells are mixed together, rabbit serum as a source of complement is added then lysis due to presence or absence of antibodies in the recipient specific for the donor cells is detected. The cross-match test is an important component of immediate pre-transplant testing for all organ transplants and is well-known as the microlymphocytotoxicity test. An improved form of this test was also used to screen patients' sera for HLA antibodies and to determine specificity. These modifications were the bases of HLA antibody screening for approximately three decades then has been substituted in recent years with extra sensitive and reproducible assays of antibody activity. The development of HLA antibody testing and the related laboratory and clinical matters that have risen with the use of this new technology forms the basis of this review. Although renal transplantation is the base for many of the lessons we have learned by means of the new methods of antibody detection like flowcytometry and Luminex based HLA antibody detection, they are similarly used in solid organ transplantation.

3.2.1a Lymphocyte cell separation Method:

Blood sample collected in 10 ml sodium heparin tube and mixed well gently. Take 3 ml ficoll hypaque (HistoPaque-1083) in 15 ml centrifuge tube. Carefully layer slowly 10 ml blood without disturbing ficoll hypaque solution, after Centrifuge for 20 minutes at room temperature, 180 x g, you will then see a thin cloudy layer at the serum/HistoPaque interface (this is the "buffy coat"/mononuclear cells layer), carefully remove and discard the top serum layer, then collect the buffy coat thin layer (avoiding the HistoPaque underneath), collect the buffy coat layer into a new 15 mL tube, Add 3 mL PBS to the buffy coat, gently resuspended cells (finger-mix), centrifuge @ room temp for 10 minutes @ 405 x g, repeat wash 3 times. After that adjust cell concentration 2.5×10^3 also check viability 80% to 100% viability cells can be used for test.

The test which trusts on the detection of complement-dependent cytotoxicity (CDC) is done in small microtiter trays. Serum samples from recipients were obtained before transplantation. Pre-transplant to detect donor-specific different types of antibodies cytotoxic cross-match (CXM) like AUTO, DTT, AHG (Anti-human globulin) was performed using CDC technique. The donor's B and T lymphocytes were isolated from peripheral blood using ficoll hypaque density gradient and patient's serum was added, and the mixture was incubated at room temperature or 18-20°C for 60 minutes, followed by a 120-minute incubation with addition of rabbit complement in order to detect any cytotoxic antibody activity against donor cells. Target cell lysis was determined by acridine orange and ethidium bromide dye. The CXM test was interpreted as positive when more than 20% of donor lymphocytes were lysed in excess of the baseline rate.

If the CDC test was positive, the recipient's serum was treated with dithiothreitol (DTT) for 30 minutes to act as a reducing agent to inactivate immunoglobulin M (IgM) antibodies, and then test was subsequently repeated. A negative CXM after DTT reduction was indicative of the presence of IgM antibodies, while a positive CXM in spite of DTT treatment indicated the presence of immunoglobulin G (IgG) antibodies.

Figure 3.4 lymphocyte cress match

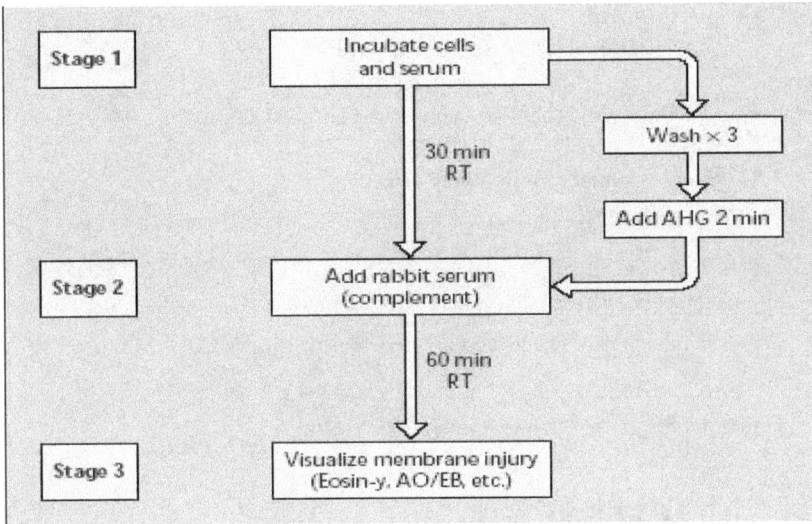

Figure 3.5 CDC cross-match result in live-green cell and dead red cells

CDC-based assays

NIH extended incubation & washes CDC:

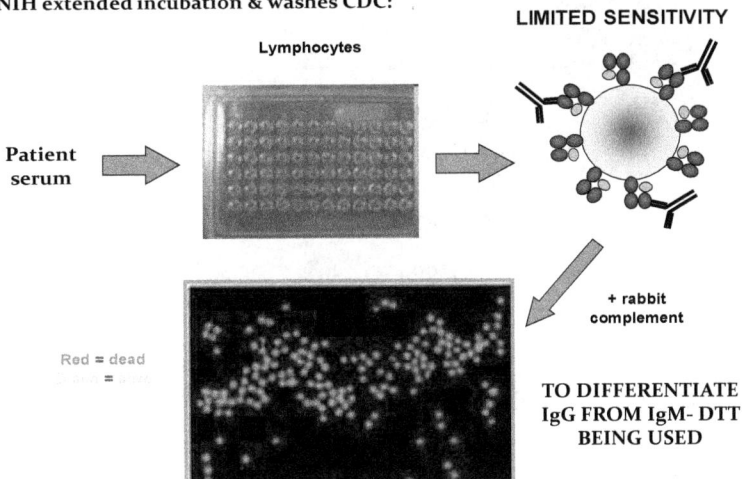

Lymphocytes

LIMITED SENSITIVITY

Patient serum

Red = dead

+ rabbit complement

TO DIFFERENTIATE IgG FROM IgM- DTT BEING USED

Test scoring 1 to 20 % dead cells- 2+ score-Negative

20-40 % dead cells – 4+ score-weak positive

40-60 % dead cells – 6+ score-positive

60-80 % dead cells – 8+ score-strong positive

3.2.2 Flow-cytometry for antibody detection

The flowcytometry lymphocyte cross-match (FCXM) is a standard technique to assess the compatibility of potential kidney transplant recipients and donors. Positive FCXM has important prognostic implication even when CDCXM is negative. So positive FCXM should not normally be dismissed as "overly sensitive" when CDCXM is negative

Figure 3.6 Flowcytometry cross-match test setup

FCM Test set-up

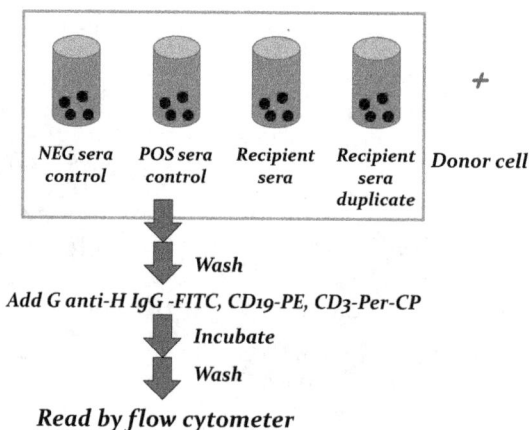

NEG sera control   POS sera control   Recipient sera   Recipient sera duplicate   Donor cell

Wash

Add G anti-H IgG -FITC, CD19-PE, CD3-Per-CP

Incubate

Wash

Read by flow cytometer

For the FCXM, 50 µl of a 2.5×10^3 cells/ml donor cell suspension was mixed with 50 µl of appropriate test and control sera. Samples were incubated for 20 min at 4°C then centrifuged and washed three times with cold phosphate-buffered saline. Fluorescence-labeled antibodies (10 µl anti-CD3 PerCP, 10 µl anti-CD19 phycoerythrin, and 100 µl of a working dilution of anti-human IgG F[ab] ' FITC) were added. After a 20-min dark incubation, two wash steps with phosphate-buffered saline were performed, and lymphocytes were resuspended in 500 μl phosphate-buffered saline with 0.05% sodium azide and transferred into tubes for analysis. Three-color flow cytometric analysis was performed with a FACSCalibur instrument (BD Biosciences, NJ). Lymphocytes were gated on the basis of their forward and side-scatter characteristics. With a scale that expressed staining intensity as a linear channel value (0 to 1024), median channel fluorescence for anti-human IgG F (ab) ' FITC was quantified on CD3+ T cells and CD19+ B cells.

Figure 3.7 Flow-cytometry: FACSCalibur

BD FACScalibur

Gating cell populations by type of fluorescence

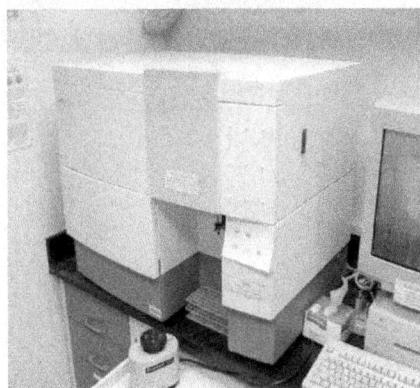
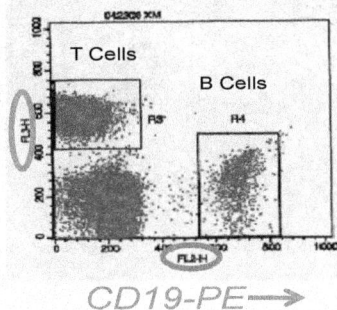

Figure 3.8 Flowcytometry crossmatch test result positive and negative control and test

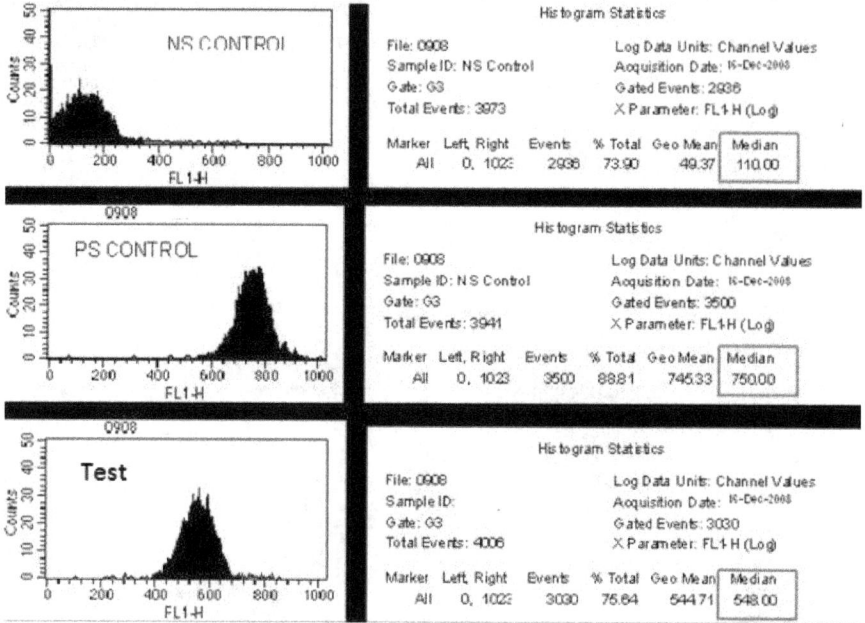

A positive flow cytometry cross-match was identified when the sample median fluorescence intensity was exceeded that of negative control values by 3 SD. SD was derived by performing negative control FCXM with sera from 12 AB-negative non-transfused males and also lymphocytes from 25 healthy donors to check the quality of control. A positive T cell FCXM and a positive B cell FCXM signified median channel shift values of ≥ 50 and ≥ 100, in that order

Pitfalls of Flow Cytometry Cross-matching

· Too sensitive

· Detection of low titer and non-complement fixing antibodies of little or clinical relevance???

· Would inappropriately deny a patient access to transplantation

· Does not reliably predict poor clinical outcomes

3.2.3 Luminex platform for HLA antibody detection

HLA antigens are polymorphic proteins expressed on donor kidney allograft endothelium and are important targets for recipient immune recognition. HLA antibodies are hazard factors for acute and chronic rejection and allograft loss. Solid-phase immunoassays for HLA antibody detection signify a major advance in sensitivity and specificity batter then cell-based methods and are generally used in organ allocation and pre-transplant risk assessment. Post-transplant, development of de-novo donor-specific HLA antibodies and/or increase in donor-specific antibodies from pre-transplant levels are associated with adversarial outcomes. Although single antigen bead assays have permitted sensitive detection of recipient HLA antibodies and their specificities, a number of explanatory considerations necessity be appreciated to understand test results in clinical and research situations. The study is relevant for clinicians thoughtful for transplant patients, discusses the technical aspects of single-antigen bead assays, emphasizes their quantitative limitations, and explores the utility of HLA antibody testing in identifying and managing important pre- and post-transplant clinical results.

For HLA antibody detection test was performed in round bottom Elisa plate, 5ul LABScreen beads incubated with 20 ul with test and control sera at 20-25° C in dark for 30 minutes with gentle shaking. After that washed three times with wash buffer. Then dilute 1ul per test of 100X PE-conjugated anti-human IgG with 99 ul of 1X wash buffer.

Add 100 ul of this diluted PE and incubate for 30 minutes at 20-25° C with gentle shaking. After this give 2 washes and resuspended in 80 ul 1X Phosphate buffer saline (PBS). And proceed to data acquisition and analysis by Fusion software (LAB Screen; One Lambda)

Figure 3.9 Luminex machine

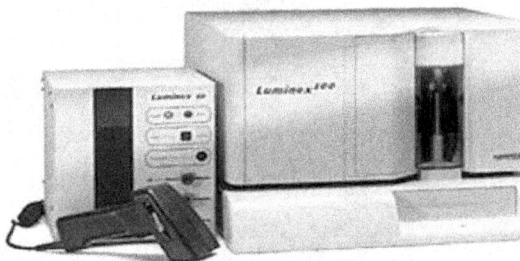

Single Antigen Beads:

Figure 3.10 HLA single antigen bead

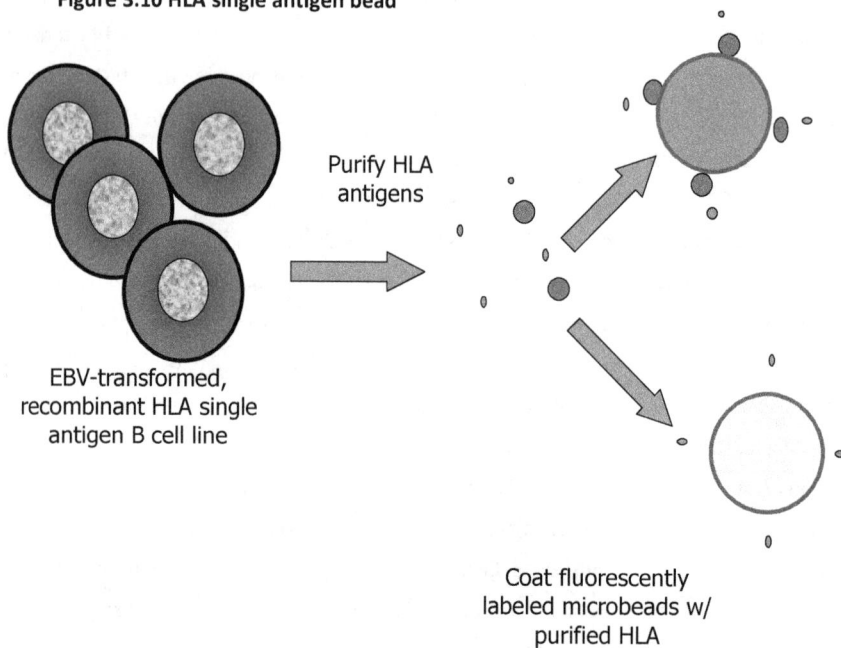

Purify HLA antigens

EBV-transformed, recombinant HLA single antigen B cell line

Coat fluorescently labeled microbeads w/ purified HLA

Figure 3.11 Leasers measure the size and fluorescence intensity of bead

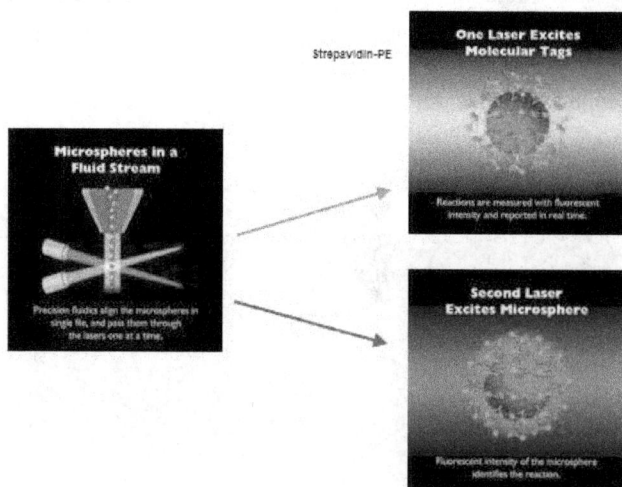

Strepavidin-PE

Microspheres in a Fluid Stream

Precision fluidics align the microspheres in single file, and pass them through the lasers one at a time.

One Laser Excites Molecular Tags

Reactions are measured with fluorescent intensity and reported in real time.

Second Laser Excites Microsphere

Fluorescent intensity of the microsphere identifies the reaction.

Figure 3.11 Leasers measure the size and fluorescence intensity of bead

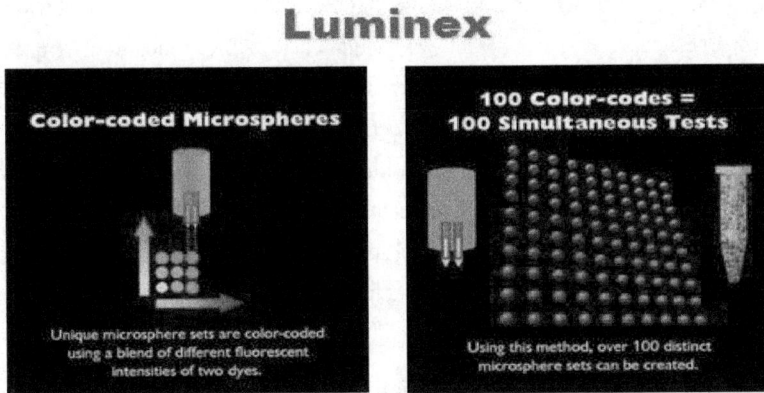

Figure 3.12 single antigen results by software

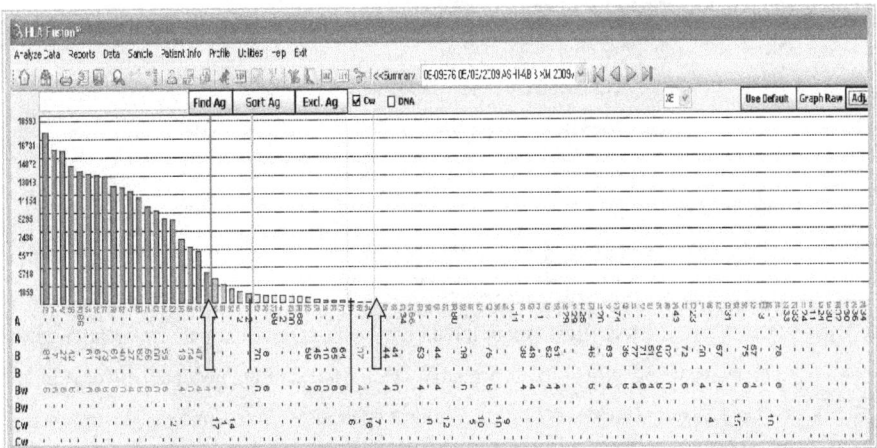

Thresholds used to define Strong, Moderate, Weak HLA antibodiesThresholds used to define Strong, Moderate, Weak HLA antibodies

Thresholds vary from one lab to another but there is good agreement on the presence/ absence of strong/moderate antibodies

Recipient sera were screened for class I and class II HLA Donor specific Antibody (DSA) through the use of single HLA antigen-charged polystyrene beads according to the

48

manufacturer's instructions (LAB Screen; One Lambda, Canoga Park, CA) utilizing a multichannel flow array (Luminex, Austin, TX), and identified via Fusion software (LAB Screen; One Lambda). Patient serum was monitored for DSA at months 1, 3, 6, 9, and 12 post-transplant, every 6 months thereafter, monitored/diagnosed for graft dysfunction or rejection. A positive de-novo DSA was defined as a new antibody not present before transplant with donor specificity and Mean fluorescence intensity (MFI) of greater than 1000 is cut off in our center. For both pre-transplant and post-transplant DSA, only those at an MFI greater than 1000 were considered. Anabel to do virtual cross-match helps to predict cross-match in sensitized patients and in diseases donor transplantation save money and time.

Advantages of Virtual Cross-match

- Adds precision to actual cross-match
- ~8% of flow cross matches false-positive –unnecessary exclusion
- ~7% of flow cross matches fail to detect DSA –risk to the patient
- Permits assessment of cross-match compatibility without access to donor tissue
- Import organs for sensitized patients
- Permits national paired exchange
- Improves allocation efficiency
- Better access for sensitized patients

3.3 Infection detection

Infections are a common reason for morbidity and mortality after transplantation, and infections rank second as the reason for death in patients with allograft function (Ko KS, 1994). The rate of first infections in the early 3 years after kidney transplantation is 45.0 per 100 patient-years of follow-up, as probable using Medicare claims data collected by the U.S. Renal Data System (Snyder JJ, 2009). With the pretransplant screening of donor and recipient, vaccination, and post-transplant surveillance and prophylaxis, the influence of infections may be reduced.

Post-transplant infections might follow an expected pattern concerning timing after transplant (Fishman JA, 2007). The modern paradigm has noted that early infections (within the first month) are more likely to be the reason for nosocomially acquired pathogens, surgical issues, and maybe donor-derived infections. Opportunistic pathogens happen later, frequently during the subsequent 5 months, reflecting the larger impact of immunosuppressive therapies. Late infections might be secondary to opportunistic pathogens or conventional ones; opportunistic pathogens are more often seen in patients who require greater immunosuppression or who have specific environmental contacts. It is important to note that though this timeline of infections is a helpful preliminary point, the pattern and timing of infections may be significantly changed by the choice of immunosuppressive agents that may affect the state of immunosuppression at different time points, in addition to the choice and duration of antimicrobial prophylactic agents.

3.3.1 Culture and sensitivity for bacterial and fungal infection

Patient blood, body fluids, and urine samples were cultured in a specifically selected medium using standard methods for bacterial and fungal infections detection. The most common growth media used for microorganisms are nutrient broths, nutrient agar plate, and MacConkey agar plate or Sabouraud agar culture medium. Selective and special media were used for the growth of only selected microorganisms. Differential media or indicator media distinguish one microorganism type from another growing on the same media. Positive samples are reported as a colony count and sensitivity of each organism.

3.3.2 Infection detection using real-time PCR

· DNA/RNA was isolated from patient's blood and urine by using standard DNA isolation kits.

· Setup the PCR test reaction and conditions for amplification of the DNA/RNA was carried out using the Qiagen kit.

Viral Detection

Procedure

DNA/RNA isolation [Hepatitis- B & C, Cytomegalovirus, BK virus, Epstein Bar virus]

· The DSP Virus Kit (QIAGEN) was validated for viral nucleic acid purification from human plasma or urine. Carry out the viral DNA/RNA purification according to the instructions in the *DSP Virus Kit.*

· Desired number of PCR tubes and reagents were isolated into the adapters of the cooling block.

· The internal control was added to the master mix.

· The reaction mix contained all of the components needed for PCR except the sample.

· Add standards and samples as per kit literature (Artus kit).

· Place assay set-up plate into Rotor Gene-Q and set PCR temperature profile
   (Amplification) according to kit literature.

· Data was analyzed using the (Artus kit software), Delta RUN Vs Cycles graph is obtained through Rotor Gene-Q software. Pathogen detection was detected in Green [FAM] channel. Positive results were reported in IU/ml or Copies/ml.

This method was used to detect all viral infections detection and treatment response measurement for CMV, BKV, EBV, HCV, and HBsAg

Figure 3.13 Real-time PCR amplification cycles

• Fluorescence-based detection of amplification

• Logarithmic amplification of a specific DNA segment by a thermocyclic reaction

• Monitor amplification of product in real-time

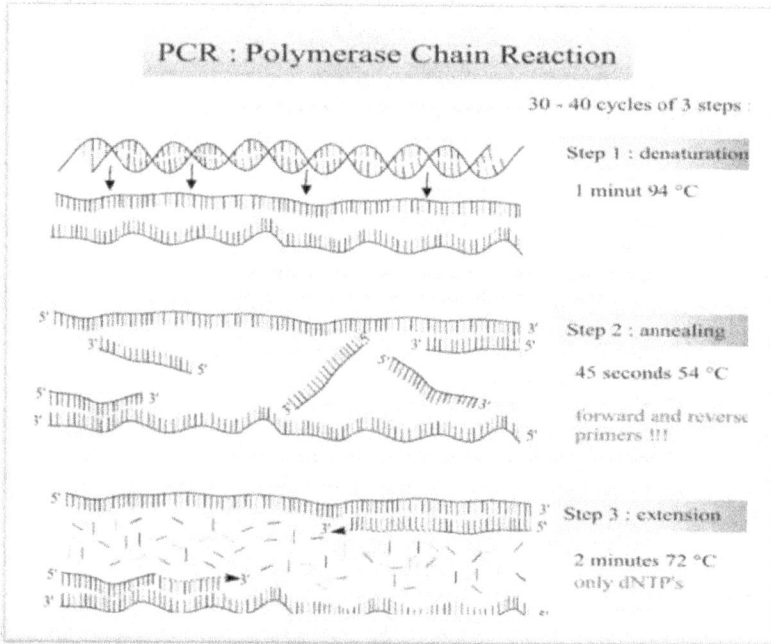

PCR : Polymerase Chain Reaction

30 - 40 cycles of 3 steps :

Step 1 : denaturation
1 minut 94 °C

Step 2 : annealing
45 seconds 54 °C
forward and reverse primers !!!

Step 3 : extension
2 minutes 72 °C
only dNTP's

- Fluorescence-based detection of amplification
- Logarithmic amplification of a specific DNA segment by a thermocyclic reaction
- Monitor amplification of product in real-time

Though infections continue a significant cause of morbidity and mortality after transplantation, better prophylactic, diagnostic, and treatment strategies have decreased the negative effect of infection on transplant outcomes. Ongoing care to infection prevention beginning before transplantation, as well as enhanced surveillance for infections, must be maintained in all patients being considered for transplantation.

Chapter 4

Results and Discussion

Chapter-4

Results and discussion

Studies over the last decade have established the role of post transplantation human leukocyte antigen (HLA) antibodies. Antibody-mediated rejection has been recognized as the leading cause of graft dysfunction and DSA (donor specific antibodies) are strongly associated with and may be a cause of allograft loss[Terasaki PI ,2008, Everly MJ ,2009] in kidney transplantation[Halloran PF,2014,Thaunat O,2016]. DSAs identified before kidney transplant can cause early rejection, such as hyperacute rejection, accelerated acute rejection and early acute antibody-mediated rejection [Sellares J-2012, Djamali A-2014]. Some studies in primates have proved that, if left untreated, an immunologic reaction starting with DSA formation will lead to chronic rejection of the allograft[Lee PC -2009, Hidalgo LG-2009]. Denovo DSA (dnDSA) formation of antibodies against donor HLA has been recognized as the risk factors for high HLA mismatches, inadequate immunosuppression and non-adherence, and graft inflammation, such as viral infection, cellular rejection, or ischemia injury which can increase graft immunogenicity[Guidicelli G-2016,Wiebe C-2012]. Denovo DSAs are predominantly directed to donor HLA class II mismatches and usually occur during the first year of kidney transplant, but they can appear anytime, even several years later[Guidicelli G-2016,Wiebe C-2012]. They have been reported to be as frequent as 15-25% in 5 years post-transplant patients [Wiebe C1-2013]. These antibodies have been reported towards both Class I and Class II antigens[Lionaki S-2013, Kim JJ-2014] Antibodies detected in conjunction with other class I and class II antibodies were associated with significantly reduced graft survival. Importantly, Antibody mediated rejection and graft loss did not occur in patients with low levels of DQ-only antibodies; however, the role of DQ DSA alone is not well studied. This study deals with the DQ DSA incidence and actual 5-year post graft outcomes extensively.

Pre-transplant cross-matches test of all patients was negative. HLA typing was carried out in patients and donor pre-transplant. Sequence specific primers [SSP] and Sequence specific oligo nucleotide [SSO] were used. Luminex-200 platform was used for HLA antibodies screening along with standard CDC, flowcytometry cross match.

Determination of post-transplant DSA

Recipient sera were screened for class I and class II HLA DSA through the use of single HLA antigen-charged polystyrene beads according to the manufacturer's instructions (LAB Screen; One Lambda, Canoga Park, CA) utilizing a multichannel flow array (Luminex, Austin, TX), and identified via Fusion software (LAB Screen; One Lambda). Patient serum was monitored for DSA at 1, 3, 6, 9, and 12 month post-transplant, every 6 months thereafter to monitor/diagnose for graft dysfunction or rejection. A positive de novo DSA was defined as a new antibody, not present before transplant, with donor specificity and a MFI of greater than 1000, which is at the lowest limit of detection by a flow cytometric crossmatch in our center. For both pre-transplant and post-transplant DSA, only those at a MFI greater than 1000 were considered.

Strength of DSA were defined as the following; weak 1000–4000 MFI, moderate >4000–8000 MFI, strong >8000–15,000 MFI, and very strong >15,000 MFI. In our system, 4000 MFI is the approximate lower limit of a positive B-cell flow cross match, while 8000 and greater MFI antibodies are associated with increasingly positive AHG cytotoxicity cross matches. Peak-MFI DSA was defined as the highest MFI of a single DSA in each individual recipient. The goal of the study is to correlate the presence of class-I and class-II antibodies with rejection episodes in kidney transplantation. Kidney transplantation is a curative therapy for hundreds of thousands of patients with end-stage organ failure. The long-term results have not much improved, and approximately half of transplant recipients will lose their allografts by 10 years after transplant. One of the main challenges in clinical transplantation is antibody-mediated rejection (AMR) initiated by anti-donor HLA antibodies. AMR is significantly associated with graft loss. The role of alloantibodies against HLA is becoming increasingly documented as critical in the pathogenesis of acute and chronic renal allograft outcomes. The antigenic targets, the machines of T and B cell activation that result in the making of antibody, the complement cascade, methods of antibody detection, and the evidence that alloantibody-mediated mechanisms are active in acute and chronic rejection. Antibody-mediated rejection (AMR) postures a major and constant challenge for long term graft survival in kidney transplantation.

This study aimed to evaluate clinical outcomes and identify poor prognostic factors in the renal transplant at the institute of kidney diseases and research center (IKDRC), Ahmedabad. In our study, 370 patients transplanted in 2013were enrolled and followed up for five years. During this period all patients were monitored for HLA antibody, infections and also any

53

other adverse event for transplant outcome. Immunosuppressive medication for each patient was an individualized prescription of drugs that also depends on the immunological risk involved in pre and post-transplant period; majority of patients received two or three drugs out of this list Calcineurin Inhibitors (Cyclosporine and Tacrolimus), Intravenous Ig, Polyclonal Antithymocyte Globulin, Antimetabolites (mycophenolate) Rituximab, a Monoclonal Antibody that targets CD20, Complement Inhibition (Eculizumab), Cytokine Inhibition (corticosteroids and Basiliximab). Also, all patients are immunized against Hepatitis B and pneumococcal infection during pre-transplant dialysis period and post-transplant CMV prophylaxis drugs are prescribed to protect from CMV infection because first three-month patients are given more immunosuppressive medication, so there are more chances of infections.

Majority of recipients were male, and females as donors either mothers or wives, so gender bias has been discussed in part-I; also in this study group most of the recipients were between 20 to 50 years age group and common diseases were chronic glomerulonephritis, hypertension, diabetes and others also discussed. After considering all factors, the transplant outcome is analysed in this study group. Importance of HLA match can be overcome by advance immunosuppressive drugs but antibody against mismatch antigens remains a major problem. Antibody against donor mismatch antigen called donor-specific antibody is contraindicated in kidney transplantation and inferior graft outcome. Denovo DSA leading to AMR may result in acute or chronic graft damage and in long term graft loss. After six years follow-up, 89.1% is graft survival, the rejection rate is 24.8%, and graft lost 10.8%, lost to follow-up 16.7%, de-novo DSA-17.6 %, non-DSA 15.1 % and infection rate 13.5 %.In DSA group those who were class I positive, dnDSA graft survival is 83.3%, class II positive group either DR or DQ or both dnDSA had 75.8% graft survival which is inferior to class I DSA. In both class I & II dnDSA positive group had 71.4 % graft survival. We have also observed that DQ antibody are more frequent and harder to remove with treatment. We have reported in a study of 644 patients showingthat those who develop de-novo DQ alone or with DR or class I antibody, 18% of patient lost graft after five years[V. Trivedi, 2018]. In this group mean fluorescence intensity (MFI) of DSA was more than 10,000. Most of the papers are considering A, B and DR antigens matching, the role of DQ antigen was not clear. Our study clearly shows that DQ antigen matching is important in transplant outcome.

Factors affecting transplant outcome: Renal failure may arise as a complication of many diseases such as diabetes, hypertension and vascular disease and is affected by several factors including age and ethnicity. End-stage renal disease (ESRD) is an advanced form of CRF where renal function is declined to 10% of normal before initiation of dialysis or renal transplantation. Renal transplantation is the only treatment recommended for ESRD. Therapeutic and prognostic heterogeneity of ESRD is currently not possible to predict. Most of the time inadequate immunosuppression may result in causation and progression of ESRD resulting in rejection. The redundancy of immune system suggests the existence of many other molecular pathways with their resident genes causing an effector response and contributing towards the heterogeneity of the complex failure leading to graft rejection. The research work embodied in this thesis is outlined in the following points.

1) Common causes of CKD

2) Gender bias

3) Age of recipient and donor

4) Human leukocyte antigen (HLA) and ABO blood group antigen in transplant

5) Donor specific antibodies through CDC and flow XM.

6) Single antigen detection- Luminex.

7) Role of sensitization

8) Rejection in kidney transplantation

9) Viral infection in kidney transplantation.

4.1-Common causes of CKD

Chronic kidney disease prevalence is about 10% of the world's population. Due to lack of exact national data collection, the occurrence of CKD in **India** is not clear. Studies have estimated that the number of new patients diagnosed with ESRD who are continuing on dialysis or transplantation is over 100,000 per year. This number underestimates the true load of kidney disease in our country given the disparity in access to health care between urban and rural populations, due to inequalities in wealth and literacy. The most common causes of kidney disease in India in men and women are diabetes and hypertension. (S.chandra Das, 2017). Certain conditions are affecting the kidneys that occur with more incidence in women -

for example, urinary tract infections that lead to infection and scarring of the kidneys, autoimmune diseases, Rheumatoid Arthritis, and Systemic Lupus Erythematous.

Chart- 4.1

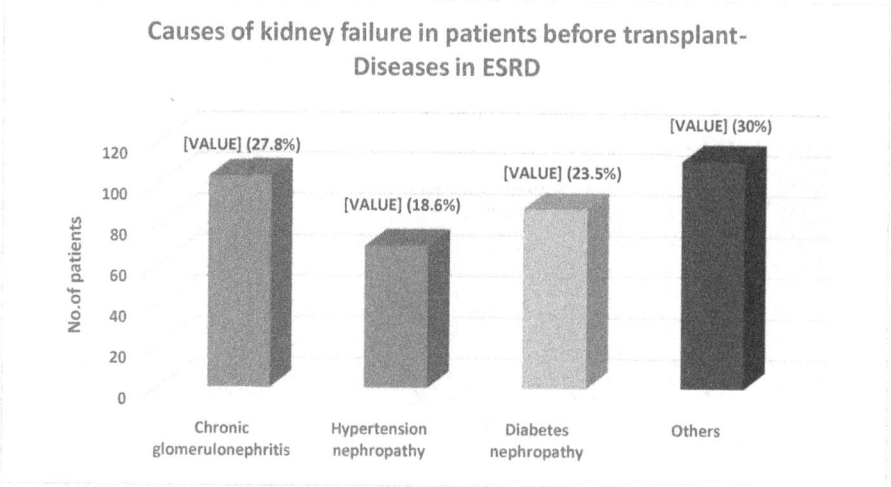

Causes of kidney failure in patients before transplant-Diseases in ESRD

Table -4.1 Causes of kidney failure in patients before transplant-Diseases in ESRD

Disease	N (%)
Chronic glomerulonephritis	103 (27.8%)
Hypertension nephropathy	69 (18.6%)
Diabetes nephropathy	87 (23.5%)
Others	111(30%)

N=number.

In our study 370 patients underwent the renal transplant in 2013. The common causes of CKD found in our study populations are chronic glomerulonephritis in 27.83%, Hypertension in 16.64%, Diabetes nephropathy in 23.51% patients, and Lupus, obstructive uropathy, Alport, FSGS, IgA nephropathy in rest of the patients.

Table-4.2 Master chart

HLA MATCH	TOTAL PT (370)	GRAFT SURVIVAL = 89.1%	REJECTION Biopsy AMR = 24.8%	GRAFT LOST =10.8%	LOST FOLLOW UP =16.7%	DSA = 17.6%	NDSA= 15.1%	INFECTION =13.5 %	2013	2014	2015	2016	2017	2018
0	17	17[100%]	5	0	3	2	2	1 HCV	0	1	1	0	0	1
1	32	29[90.6%]	9	3	9	5	5	7	4	2 +1	1+1	0	1	2
2	38	32[84.2%]	9	7	6	9	6	6	1	1	1	3+ 1	3	2+1
3	23	21[91.3%]	7	2	7	5	4	1 HCV	1	2	3	1 + 1	0	1
4	17	16[94.1%]	6	1	5	2	1	1 HBV+1 CMV, BKV	1	1	2 + 1	0	1	0
5	154	143 [92.8%]	40	11	23	33	22	22	9	8 + 2	2	4 + 1	5	3
6	51	38[74.5%]	9	13	6	7	10	1 FUNGUS +4 BACT	1	2+1	1+1	1+ 4	5 + 1	2
7	22	21[95.4%]	5	1	2	0	4	4	0	2	0	0	0	1
8	5	5[100%]	1	0	0	0	1	0	0	0	0	0	0	0
9	6	6[100%]	1	0	0	2	0	1 CMV	0	0	0	0	0	0
10	5	3[60%]	0	2	1	0	1	CMV 1+AMR	1	0	0	1	0	1

Above master data table describes five years events and outcome of 370 transplanted patients in study.

1. Colum-1 HLA antigen (A,B,C,DR,DQ)
2. Colum-2 Number of patients and number of HLA match
3. Colum-3 Graft survival after six years of renal transplantation
4. Colum-4 Biopsy proven rejection
5. Colum-5 Graft loss after six years of renal transplantation
6. Colum-6 Number of patients-lost to follow-up

7. Colum-7 Donor specific antibody (DSA) after transplantation
8. Colum-8 Non donor specific antibody(NDSA) after transplantation
9. Colum-9 Infections after transplantation
10. Colum-10-15 six year follow-up

HLA matching with donors graft survival overall after six years is 89.1%, the rejection rate is 24.8%, and graft lost 10.8%, lost to follow-up 16.7%, de-novo DSA-17.5%, and non-DSA 15.1%

4.2-Gender bias:

Kidney transplantation is performed routinely as a treatment for ESRD. However, the literature shows that there is a remarkable difference between male and female distribution/ occurrence/symptoms. It is quite clear that females are mostly donors as compared to males. On the contrary recipients of organs mainly are males, hence revealing a gender bias in the distribution of male: female ratio in live related renal transplantation. They have further revealed that there are differences among western countries, some of which lack specific rules.

Table 4.3 Relationships of kidney recipients and donors enrolled in the study

Recipients	Donors	Number
Offspring and Parents		
Son	Mother	120 (32.4%)
Son	Father	39(10.5%)
Siblings		
Brother	Brother	15 (4.0%)
Brother	Sister	17 (4.6%)
Sister	Brother	3 (0.8%)
Sister	Sister	2 (0.5%)
Parents and Offspring		
Father	Son	2 (0.5%)
Mother	Son	0
Spouse		
Husband	Wife	80 (21.6%)
Wife	Husband	20 (5.4%)
Others	Kidney Paired Donation	63 (17%)
	Extended	9 (2.4%)

N=number of pairs; KPD=pairs receiving transplants via kidney paired donation

This thesis data reveals the same trend in gender.71.35% of living donors were women, whereas 90.81% of total transplants were performed in males.

In India, by law, only family members can donate a kidney in living related KT.

In Indian study (M. BAL, 2007), among the donors, there was more female than male donors (66.1 vs. 33.9%). Most of the live donations were by mothers (32.1%). In the group of spousal pairs, the highest gender disparity was observed with predominantly wives donating for their husbands (90.7% vs 9.3%). (Organ donation Gender Bias in Renal Transplantation: Are Women alone Donating Kidneys in India) complex social and economic issues are responsible for the overall gender imbalance. Treatment for chronic kidney disease emphasizes on slowing the progression of kidney damage, usually by treating the underlying cause. Chronic kidney disease can lead to end-stage kidney failure, which is fatal without artificial filtering (dialysis) or a kidney transplant. Once a patient reaches progressive stages of CKD, kidney replacement treatment will be needed. Kidney replacement therapy can be either dialysis or kidney transplantation; with transplantation offering the best health results. Studies show that women tend to have more complications with dialysis than men; as an example, the occurrence of low blood counts and poor nutritional levels appear to be higher. They may fare just as well as their male counterparts post kidney transplantation. However, the number of male patients who receive either dialysis or kidney transplantation is significantly greater than women. Studies from countries in the world, including India, indicate a disparity in the registration of women on the deceased organ donation waiting lists and longer waiting times for women on dialysis. Worldwide and in India, women tend to serve more often as kidney donors - mothers and wives are much more likely to be donors than fathers or husbands. The recurring theme here seems to be the access to kidney care and obviously, there is considerable inequality in access to care between the genders. Socio-economic, educational and psychological reasons are all likely in play. Specific gender roles are still not clearly defined in India. Women in our country today still have less access to education and so tend to be more financially dependent on men. Majority of the families, men may be the sole or major bread-winners. The family's essential to keep a male member with CKD in the work-force may be a strong factor impacting the higher probability of women serving as donors. A woman may be donating due to a feeling of obligation of the male patient or other family members. Donor and recipient pairs undergoing transplant evaluation do have to meet with a psychiatrist who will need assistance to assess these psychosocial issues; however, given the strong cultural and financial issues some families face in India, these cases are complex. The added stigma in traditional Indian society of the young unmarried woman with a chronic medical condition that carries a monetary burden and affects fertility and pregnancy can significantly affect her marriage prospects and therefore future family life.

4.3 Age of recipient and donor

Over the last decades, the emerging evidence of the benefits and safety of kidney transplant in the elderly, as well as the ageing of the overall ESRD population, has led to the patients on transplant waiting lists growing significantly older in many countries, with the largest absolute and relative increase in the 65 years or older age group (de Fijter JW. 2009) In the United States between 1997 and 2014, whereas the waiting list for KT increased from 30 000 to more than 100 000 candidates, the proportion of candidates 65 years or older has grown from 7% to over 21% (Network. OPaT. 2015). In France, this proportion increased from 2.4% in 1998 to 11.7% in 2011, with individuals 70 years or older, representing almost half of this elderly group (Mamzer-Bruneel MF 2012)

Our study also includes small numbers of elderly (above 50 years) recipients (7.8%) at Institute of kidney diseases and research center (IKDRC). It helped elderly patients to have better quality of life by following guidelines of extended criteria for a donor (ECD) try to match the age of recipient and donor along with other guidelines, life. ECD are small in numbers but increase the rate of the transplant.

Table - 4.4 Correlation of recipient ages with rejection

Age in years	Number of patients (%)	Number of patients with rejection (%)
0-18	30 (8.1%)	10 (33.3%)
19-50	311 (84.0%)	115 (36.9%)
Above 50	29 (7.8%)	13 (44.8%)
Total	370	

The table shows the Age group between 1-18 years 8.1% recipients, 19 to 50 age group 84.0% And above 50 years were 7.8% recipients however rejection rate was higher in older i.e. above 50 years age group.

4.4 Human leucocytes antigen (HLA) and ABO blood group antigen in transplant

HLA genes are located on the short arm of chromosome 6 at 6p21 position [Tilahun Alelign, 2018], on a genetic region of 4 Mbps [Tilahun Alelign, 2018]. The human immune system uses HLA's uniqueness to distinguish self from nonself. HLA is responsible for the presentation of "foreign" peptides (antigens) to the immune-competent cells. T lymphocytes recognize foreign antigens once its associations with HLA molecules. Groups of cell surface proteins encoded by genes in MHC which are recognized as HLA in humans. HLA are groups of cell surface proteins encoded by genes in MHC they are known as HLA in humans [Tilahun Alelign, 2018]. HLA genes are located on the short arm of chromosome 6 at 6p21 location [Tilahun Alelign, 2018], a genetic region of 4 Mbps [Tilahun Alelign, 2018]. The human immune system uses HLA's distinctiveness to differentiate self from nonself. HLA is responsible for the presentation of "foreign" peptides (antigens) to the immune-competent cells. T lymphocytes identify foreign antigens when it combines with HLA molecules. Based on the construction of the antigens produced and function, two classes of HLA, HLA class I and class II. Studies have clustered the genes into three separate loci, that is, HLA class I, class III, and class II. Class I histocompatibility antigens (HLA-A, B, and C) are expressed on all cells, and class II histocompatibility antigens (HLA-DP, DQ, and DR) are expressed on antigen-presenting cells (B-cells, macrophages, dendritic cells, Langerhans cells, and capillary endothelium). Histocompatibility antigens are inherited from both parents as MHC haplotypes. It is composed of 5 to 8 exons and ranges in size from 4 to 17 kb. HLA includes numerous loci closely linked, and for each of these loci involves numerous alleles, 40 to 60 alleles per locus that control the production of their equivalent antigens. HLA mismatches might happen at antigenic or allelic levels is characterized by amino acid substitutions in both peptide-binding and T-cell recognition regions, the latter is characterized by amino acid substitutions in the peptide-binding regions. Kidney transplantation is associated with a 68% lesser risk of death than dialysis. Kidney donors might be either deceased or living sources. The first successful kidney transplantation was performed between identical twins in Boston in 1954.The ABO system antigens are important blood cell antigens in transfusion. These antigens are complex carbohydrates (polysaccharides) expressed on the surface of RBCs and numerous other cell types i.e. vascular endothelium. In spite of appropriate ABO antigen cross-matching, patients would experience transfusion reactions once they receive multiple transfusions. An ABO-incompatible organ transplant causes hyper-acute rejection due to the presence of preformed hemagglutinin A and/or B antibodies to non-self A or B antigens. ABO-incompatible transplants are done if the matched donor is not available, but it is more expensive and risky.

HLA matching both at class I and II loci is well established and practiced for each donor-recipient that has contributed significantly to better transplant result worldwide even in the cyclosporine era. Swap donor program is also popular to get better matched (HLA, blood group or age) donor HLA typing is a crucial test in renal transplantation, as recognition of foreign HLA by recipient T lymphocytes would activate an immune response. T lymphocyte activation initiates a cascade of mediators that direct against the immune system of the allograft [Moh. Mahdi Althaf, 2017]. HLA laboratories presently perform serologic as well as molecular typing methods (Low, High resolution).

In Our study group for all patients and donors, HLA typing was carried out using the molecular method through Sequence-specific primers (SSP) or sequence-specific oligonucleotide probe (SSO) low resolution typing for HLA A, B, C, DR and DQ locus. All mismatches were identified to find DSA in post-transplant monitoring. In living-related transplant, most of the recipients had only one donor from family so there was no choice for better match donor. If the recipient develops de-novo DP antibody, then DP typing of donor is done retrospectively to know whether these antibodies are DSA or not? So, further treatment can be planned more carefully.

HLA-DQ antigen is not given importance but we have demonstrated in our study (Trivedi V.B - 2018) that de-novo DQ antibodies alone can be responsible for poor long-term graft outcome. Total 644 patients studied for five years. Donor-specific antibodies (DSA) have proved a well-established biomarker predicting antibody against the human leukocyte antigen (HLA)-A, -B, and -DR loci. It has detrimental effect on renal allograft outcomes including high incidence of antibody-mediated rejection, graft dysfunction, inferior graft survival and poor transplant outcomes. Inadequate data is available describing the incidence and impact of *denovo* HLA-DQ antibodies. 644 renal transplant recipients without pre-transplant donor-specific antibodies over the period of four years from the western part of India were examined. 23% (157/644) patients developed donor-specific antibodies, in which 17.8% (28) had a HLA-class I and 82.6% (129) had class II antibodies.55.8% (72) class II positive patients developed denovo DQ antibodies. The mean of serum creatinine and proteinuria was significantly higher in HLA-DQ antibodies developed patients than those without antibodies.18.05% (13/72) denovo positive patients rejected grafts. The study is conclusive that the donor-specific HLA-DQ antibodies were the most common type detected and these antibodies may contribute to poor graft outcomes.

CHART-4.2 Study groups division on basis of denovo NDSA antibodies

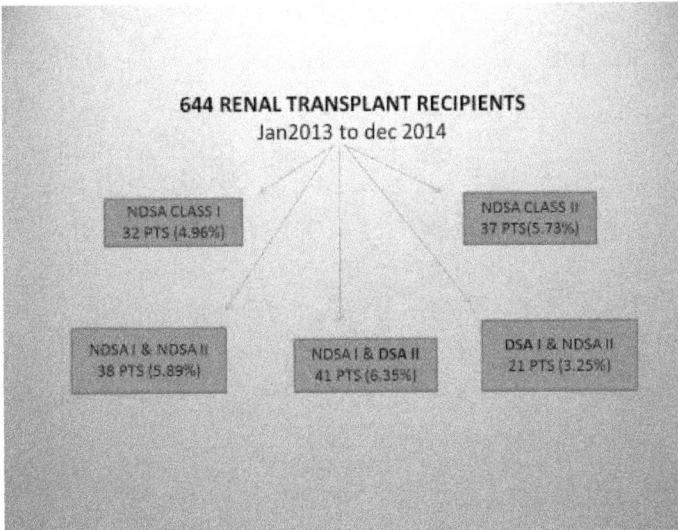

644 RENAL TRANSPLANT RECIPIENTS
Jan2013 to dec 2014

NDSA CLASS I
32 PTS (4.96%)

NDSA CLASS II
37 PTS(5.73%)

NDSA I & NDSA II
38 PTS (5.89%)

NDSA I & DSA II
41 PTS (6.35%)

DSA I & NDSA II
21 PTS (3.25%)

Above chart shows denovo NDSA antibodies. Class-I 4.9% class-II 5.73%

Class I & II 5.89%, NDSA + DSA class I & II 6.35% and 3.25%

CHART-4.3 Study groups division on basis of denovo DSA antibodies

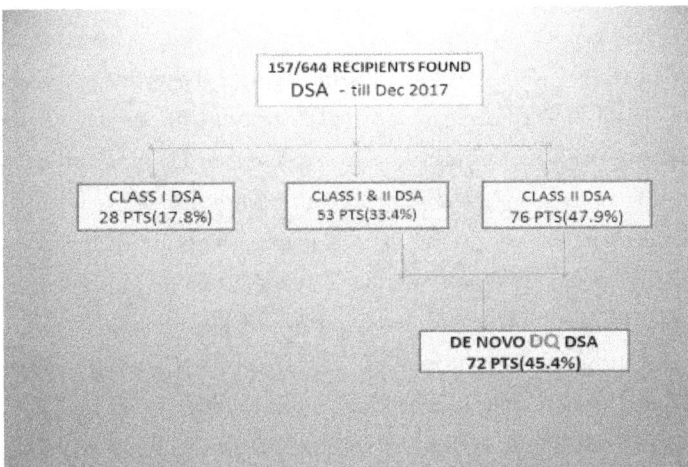

157/644 RECIPIENTS FOUND
DSA - till Dec 2017

CLASS I DSA
28 PTS(17.8%)

CLASS I & II DSA
53 PTS(33.4%)

CLASS II DSA
76 PTS(47.9%)

DE NOVO DQ DSA
72 PTS(45.4%)

Chart-2 shows denovo development of DSA antibodies. Total 157-24.3% out of those class I-17.8%, II-33.4% and both I & II -47.9% over all DQ antibodies found in 45.4%

CHART-4.4 Denovo DQ DSA antibodies vs graft outcome

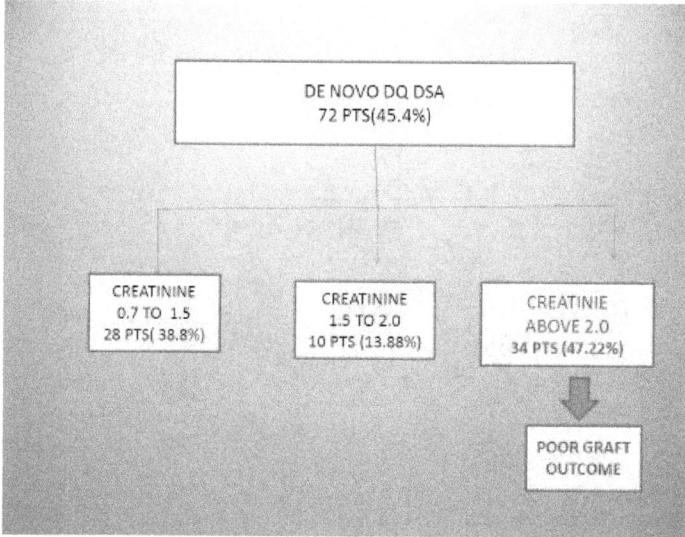

```
                    DE NOVO DQ DSA
                    72 PTS(45.4%)


   CREATININE          CREATININE          CREATINIE
   0.7 TO 1.5          1.5 TO 2.0          ABOVE 2.0
   28 PTS( 38.8%)      10 PTS (13.88%)     34 PTS (47.22%)


                                          POOR GRAFT
                                          OUTCOME
```

Chart-3 shows correlation between DQ DSA antibodies and poor graft outcome

Gradually increase in S.Creatinine value shows poor graft function in presence of DSA DQ antibodies.

Donor-specific antibodies (DSA) have proved a well-established biomarker predicting antibody against the HLA-A, -B, and -DR loci. It harms the renal allograft outcomes including a high incidence of antibody-mediated rejection, graft dysfunction, inferior graft survival, and poor transplant outcomes. Inadequate data is available describing the incidence and impact of de-novo HLA-DQ antibodies. In our study we have shown that the patients from the western part of India were transplanted and observed (paper published) that they do not have pre-transplant donor-specific antibodies. All patients were followed for over five years from the day of kidney transplant. After five years, out of 644 patients only 23% (157/644) patient's developed donor-specific antibodies, of which 17.8% (28/157) had HLA-class I and 82.6% (129/157) had class II antibodies. In class II DSA positive group 55.8%, (72/157) patients developed de-novo DQ antibodies or in addition to DQ antibody, there were class I or class II DR antibodies. The mean of serum creatinine and proteinuria were significantly higher in the patients that have developed HLA-DQ antibodies.18.05% (13/72) de-novo positive patients rejected grafts within five years. The study concludes that the donor-specific HLA-DQ antibodies are the most common type detected and these antibodies may contribute to poor graft outcomes.

Data from the United Network for Organ Sharing (UNOS) registry further highlighted the implication of paying consideration to having the minimum number of mismatches. They looked at quantifying the risk of transplanted graft failure with HLA mismatch in patients who had their first kidney allografts from deceased donors. This study shown that having six HLA mismatches translated to a 64% higher risk whereas the risk was down to 13% with just one HLA mismatch. Also, these results were independent of the locus [Williams RC, 2016]. Another study identified seven specific HLA mismatch combinations that were associated with decreased renal allograft survival [Doxiadis II, 1996]. In recent times, the HLA mismatching in deceased donor kidney transplants is of lesser significance due to the use of more potent immunosuppression and improved identification of non-immunological determinants of transplantation [Su X, Zenios SA, 2004]. However, HLA matching continues to have a significant impact on allograft survival. Allelic variations found in the promoters/exons/ un-translated regions of the genes often results in the heterogeneity of the expression profile of the respective genes. This type of allelic variation that triggers variables expression level constitutes the "high, moderate and low producing genotype" depending on their effects on the transcription level of the concerned Genes. So, the expression level of these factors, up to a certain level is predetermined in each individual and hence the genotypic profile might provide a significant guideline for evaluating effective levels of immunosuppressive agents; added required medications HLA mismatch results into both T-cells mediated immune responses that stimulate cytokine production and sooner antibody-mediated cell cytotoxicity. In spite of having a matched HLA profile among ESRD patients and their corresponding allograft donors, chances of allograft rejection have been noticed in the post-transplantation situation which might be due to effector responses of numerous other molecular pathways with their resident genes.

Population studies carried out over the decades have identified a long list of human diseases that are significantly more common amongst individuals that carry particular HLA alleles. For example, 90% of Caucasian patients with ankylosing spondylitis carry particular class I HLA alleles e.g., HLA-B*27:02, HLA-B*27:05 (Reveille, 2006). Narcolepsy, a brain disorder characterized by sleep abnormality and falling attacks (cataplexy), is an explanatory example the DQB1*06:02 alleles (Mignot et al., 1994). In type-I diabetes mellitus, more than 90% of patients carry either HLA-DRB1*03/DQB1*02:01 or HLA-DRB1*04/DQB1*03:02 gene haplotypes likened to only 40% of controls (Erlich et al., 2008). Rheumatoid arthritis (RA) is an additional emblematic HLA class II-associated disease (reviewed in Holoshitz, 2010). Approximately 90% of Caucasian seropositive RA patients carry one or two HLA-DRB1 alleles (e.g., DRB1*04:01, DRB1*04:04, DRB1*04:05, DRB1*01:01, and a few others) that code for a sequence motif in the DRβ chain called "shared epitope" (SE).

4.5 Donor specific antibodies through CDC, Flow XM

Study group

In this study we have used all three tests for screening the preformed and de-novo antibodies and its relevance in transplantation. Pre-transplant of all 370 recipients were negative for CDC, FCM, and HLA antibody screen tests. All recipients were a monitor for five years for de-novo anti-HLA antibodies (HLAab) at a regular interval or if there is the rise of serum creatinine for some reason like infection, rejection, drug toxicity or any other reason.

4.5.1 Complement-dependent cytotoxicity (CDC) crossmatch

The first clinically documented antibody-mediated syndrome in the current era of transplantation was described in 1968 in the landmark paper of Terasaki and Patel (Patel R, Terasaki PI, 1969). In a study of 225 renal transplant patients, in which 32 had primary non-functional graft, 24 of 32 had evidence of a circulating factor in recipient serum that caused CDC of donor lymphocytes, compared with only six of 193 with primary graft function who had same factor demonstrable. The initial non-functioning graft recognized as hyperacute rejection in which catastrophic intravascular thrombosis and necrosis are almost instant after graft reperfusion. The circulating factor described is recognized to be an anti-donor antibody, and in most cases it is anti-HLA antibody. The CDC assay used in the study, with little modification has formed the basis for the T cell cross-match. Recognition of this antibody-mediated rejection and the ability of the T cell cross-match to forecast its incidence if positive have eliminated the entity of hyperacute rejection in modern transplantation. Studies demonstrating the clinical relevance of anti-HLA antibodies have been published (Patel R, Terasaki PI, 1969) Because of the application of Complement Dependent Cytotoxicity test (CDC) cross-match testing in histocompatibility laboratories, hyperacute rejection has become a rare event. The cytotoxic assay was implemented because during the test pre-transplantation it was indicated that recipients with DSA had higher rates of allograft failure due to hyperacute rejection as well as primary failure [Patel R, Terasaki PI, 1969, Stiller CR, 1975]. The presence of donor-specific cytotoxic antibodies displayed as a positive cross-match was a contraindication to transplantation. Despite the clear benefits of testing T cell cytotoxic crossmatch, there was twenty percent false positive rate and a four percent false-negative rate. Therefore, it is insufficient to identify all relevant antibodies, and in addition to that, it may needlessly exclude patients from transplant. The solid-phase antibody test was used together with crossmatch results to identify those that are immunologically relevant [Gebel HM, 2003].

Similar to cytotoxic assay the complement-dependent cytotoxicity crossmatch is understood as positive if a considerable number of lymphocytes are destroyed after the incorporation of complement. This suggests that a substantial DSA has been bound to the cell surface. Complement-dependent cytotoxicity cross matches (CDC-XM) can be done for B and T lymphocytes. Sensitivity is limited if the relevant antibody is in low titers, but this can be overcome by increasing the incubation time, the use of the AHG-enhanced method as well as additional wash steps[Amos DB, 1970, Fuller TC,1997]. The complement-fixing antibody to anti-human immunoglobulin (AHG) will bind to any DSA present on lymphocytes. This upsurges the chances of activating complement and therefore raises the sensitivity of the test.

The antibodies are present in lower titers are clinically significant as a negative test has an 18% graft loss in 1 year compared to a positive test that is related with 36% [Kerman RH, 1991]. Sera that gave a positive result with CDC but a negative result with the Luminex method were retested with and without dithiothreitol (DTT) to differentiate between IgM and IgG antibodies.

4.5.2 Flow cytometry crossmatch

In 1983, Garovoy et al introduced the flow cytometry crossmatch (FCXM) assay, it was a highly sensitive cross-match technique. The FCXM assay can be done on a large number of cells (5,000- 10,000 cells) within a minute and provides an objective evaluation of patient serum antibodies to HLA-specificities of donor target cells. It detect weak positive reactions (false-negative cross matches) better than the use of a light microscope. Though, the FCXM assay has not been widely used as the standard NIH- and AHG method.

Flow cytometry cross match (FCXM) detects DSA independent of complement fixation. It exactly detects the presence or lack of IgG DSA on donor lymphocytes. In this test, recipient serum is mixed with donor lymphocytes and then tagged with a fluorochrome-conjugated anti-IgG antibody. Some antibodies with separate fluorochromes particular to B and T lymphocyte surface proteins can be added. With the use of flow-cytometry, B and T lymphocytes can be readily identified and have their DSA individually detected. Compared to complement-dependent cytotoxicity cross-match this offers greater sensitivity [Tinckam KJ, 2012].

4.6 Luminex methodology -HLA antibody detection testing

The detection of antibodies against the human leukocyte antigen (HLA) complex has become crucial in every clinical practice. The development of solid-phase assays like the Luminex permits the standardized measurement of anti-HLA antibodies (HLAab) with high sensitivity, although the relevance for some clinical settings remains a matter of debate. Principle of Luminex-based antibody detection, with two modifications that allow identifying solely complement-activating antibodies. The Luminex-based assays use polystyrene microbeads impregnated with a unique mixture of two fluorescent dyes, are simultaneously excited by a red laser at 635 nm. The emitted light can be detected at wavelengths of 660 nm (red) and 730 nm (infrared) by means of a dedicated footprint flow cytometer (Luminex®100/200™). By measuring the composition of the emission intensities for both channels, up to 100 distinct beads with a unique HLA antigen can be identified parallel. The detection of HLAab is achieved by using a secondary antibody and conjugated with the reporter fluorophore R-phycoerythrin (PE) which is excited by a green laser (532 nm) and detected at 576 nm.

Though bead-based immunoassays are approved only for qualitative assignment of HLAab specificities, numerous publications demonstrate to some extent correlations of the mean fluorescence intensity (MFI) of the detection antibody as measured in Luminex bead arrays with cross-match results using CDC or flow cytometry and clinical outcomes [Mizutani K, 2007, Vaidya S, 2008]. Nevertheless, MFI measures cannot directly be converted into antibody titers as the MFI just represents a surrogate marker for the amount of bound antibody and is affected by several factors, including antibody concentration in the serum but also density, conformation and orientation of the antigen, also by the antibody avidity toward the respective antigen Now, increasing efforts are to tailor the maintenance immunosuppressive therapy to the individual allograft recipient, based on surrogate markers for rejection and tolerance [Gillespie A, 2008]. Detection of de novo DSA by means of Luminex constitutes a suitable non-invasive biomarker to identify patients with increased risk for antibody-mediated rejection (AMR) [Liefeldt L, 2012]. When AMR occurs, monitoring of the DSA level provides to some extent a prediction of the outcome: In a series of 10 patients treated for refractory AMR with the proteasome inhibitor bortezomib the continued reduction of the strongest DSA as indicated by the MFI was predictive for improved 18-month allograft survival and reversal of AMR [Waiser J,, 2012].

These findings emphasize the versatile applications of the standard and modified Luminex assays for pretransplant risk stratification and prediction of rejection and also for monitoring of therapeutic interventions in solid-organ transplantation.

Taking all aspects mentioned into consideration, the Luminex technology is a sophisticated technique that requires interpreters with educated experience and expertise. Application of the appropriate Luminex assays allows both detections of all HLAab with high sensitivity and the exclusive recognition of those HLAab that are clinically relevant due to their complement-activating capacity. Luminex thus provides valuable information for bona fide decision making in a variety of clinical settings.

4.7 Role of sensitization

Presence of HLAab is called sensitization. Reasons for Sensitization are blood transfusion, transplantation, pregnancy (female), infection, vaccination. If a patient develops HLAab against donor's mismatch antigen is called DSA other called non-DSA. Presence of HLAab is called sensitization which is bad news for transplant.

Pre-transplant HLAab (DSA) may lead to hyperacute rejection so they are contraindicated in transplantation. Patients who develop de-novo HLAab may suffer AMR or chronic rejection so there will be poor graft outcome there for it is necessary to remove and stop production of antibodies by desensitization treatment. Different protocols followed by different center's use of Bortezomib, IVIG, and plasmapheresis.

Table-4.5- Results of Luminex antibody screening compared to Luminex SAB reactivity in the same sample

Screening results		Number of patients (%)	Single antigen bead results		
Class I	Class II	Screening test	DSA	NDSA	No HLA antibody
Pos	Neg	64 (17.3%)	12 (3.2%)	17 (4.6%)	35
Pos	Pos	41 (11.1%)	24 (6.5%)	22 (5.9%)	---
Neg	Pos	43 (11.6%)	29 (7.8%)	17 (4.6%)	
Neg	Neg	249 (67.3%)	N/A	N/A	N/A

DSA=donor specific HLA antibody; NDSA = HLA antibody present but no donor-specific antibody;

As shown in the above table in our study group, strategy for post-transplant HLAab monitoring was first screening test is advised and if screening test positive then single antigen class I & II test will be advised. 67.3% patients did not develop any HLAab while rest of patients 32.7% were positive for screening test further they were tested for single-antigen class I & II, results were analyzed for DSA and NDSA HLA antibody also Mean fluorescence intensity was noted so patients can be monitored for treatment response.

In class I test positive group 3.2% patients develop DSA and 4.6% NDSA, class II positive group 7.8% develop DSA while 4.6% NDSA for both class I & II positive group 6.5% DSA and 5.9% NDSA.

Table 4.6 Specificities and level of reactivity of de-novo HLA class I donor-specific antibodies identified post-transplant and graft outcome.

HLA antigen	MFI	S.Creatinine	Graft Outcome
B44	1296	1.06	Survive
A24	5214	1.45	Survive
A1	4517	3.42	FOLLOW UP LOST
B57	9638	12.91	Graft Lost
A11	2549	10.24	Graft Lost
B57	3398	2.22	FOLLOW UP LOST
B57	2007	1.74	Survive
A24	4098	1.27	Survive
C7	14136	0.8	Survive
A33	2705	1.36	Survive
A26	8423	0.85	Survive
B55	1536	--	EXPIRED*

MFI= mean fluorescent intensity of bead with specified antigen (if two beads had the same antigen, highest value was used); S. creatinine = serum creatinine; * death due to surgical complication
When describing tables, serum creatinine was measured at the time of antibody testing

Table -4.7 Specificities and level of reactivity of de-novo class II donor specific antibodies identified post-transplant and graft outcome.

HLA antigen	MFI	S.Creatinine	Graft Lost
DQ6	3825	1.32	FOLLOW UP LOST
DQ5	8378	12.81	Graft Lost
DQ7	1855	2.68	FOLLOW UP LOST
DR14	2207	8.6	Graft Lost
DR51	3153	1.08	Survive
DQ2	3781	5.66	Graft Lost
DQ7	1589	1.06	FOLLOW UP LOST
DQ6	1275	3.81	Survive
DQ8	9933	6.96	Graft Lost
DQ7	1948	1.33	Survive
DR52 DQ5 DR 10	3168, 1204, 1654	1.15	Survive
DQ2 DR17	5365, 1022	1.04	Survive
DQ6	1015	0.97	Survive
DQ7 DQ9	3550, 2660	1.08	Survive
DR51 DQ6	3291, 2273	0.87	Survive
DQ5	3421	1.54	Survive
DQ8	2580	1.53	Survive
DR13	3779	13.73	Graft Lost
DQ7	7114	3.04	FOLLOW UP LOST
DR51	4933	8.47	Graft Lost
DR53	1521	1.71	Survive
DQ2 DQ5	6674	7.5	Graft Lost
DQ8	4512	1.64	Survive
DQ5	2500	1.52	Survive
DQ6	2928	1.1	Survive
DR52	1933	0.83	Survive
DQ 2	2221	1.39	Survive
DQ 2	10133	0.89	Survive

Table -4.8 Specificities and level of reactivity of de-novo class I & II donor specific antibodies identified post-transplant and graft outcome.

No	ANTIGEN (Class I)	MFI	ANTIGEN (Class II)	MFI	S.Creatinine	Graft Lost
1	A32	2433	DQ7	1574	2.26	Survive
2	A24	2504	DQ8	1936	1.45	Survive
3	A26 A2	1824 7200	DQ6 DQ7 DR51	6530 1574	9.32	Graft Lost
4	C15	1030	DR51 DQ6 DR15	3987 3739 3609	2.18	FOLLOW UP LOST
5	A1	2830	DQ6 DQ7 DR15	4478, 11852, 1204	3.81	Survive
6	C15 A68	1965 1360	DQ8 DR53	8108 ,1404	1.3	FOLLOW UP LOST
7	A24 B58	5575 4063	DQ2 DQ7 DR11 DR17	1058,3119, 5039,13598	2.33	FOLLOW UP LOST
8	A2	1518	DR11 DQ7 DR8	5039 3119	0.95	Survive
9	B51 C4 C14	6581 2613 9860	DQ7	3481	12.4	Graft Lost
10	B57 A2	8518 3468	DR53 DQ2	1423 1252	4.16	FOLLOW UP LOST
11	A1 B55	3320 1113	DQ2 DQ6 DR52 DR7	4928 4515	8.14	Graft Lost
12	A24	3122	DR52	1367	2.15	Survive
13	B55	1536	DR7 DR52 DR11 DQ7 DQ9	3400 5481 3209	--	EXPIRED (Surgical)
14	A24 C5	4098	DR 1	A468	1.27	Survive
15	A1	1199	DR51 DR15 DR13 DR52	11991 6731 4901 4000	0.85	Survive
16	C7	14136	DR10	1972	0.9	Survive
17	A24	1048	DR52	1448	2.69	Survive
18	B8 CW7	1964 1343	DR52	1771	1.02	Survive
19	C7 C14	12548 11691	DR17 DR13 DR52	3078 5389	0.67	Survive
20	A1,B7	7238, 2681	DR 10	9632	7.92	Graft Lost
21	Cw7	9497	DR 4, DQ 2	9852, 8100	12.4	Graft Lost

MFI: mean fluorescent intensity of bead with specified antigen (if two beads had the same antigen, highest value was used); S. creatinine = serum creatinine; * death due to surgical complication
When describing tables, serum creatinine was measured at the time of antibody testing

Table - 4.9 HLA Luminex single antigen bead results correlated to graft survival

Single antigen bead results (Class I / Class II)=370 patients	DSA		NDSA	
	GRAFT SURVIVAL	**GRAFT LOST**	**GRAFT SURVIVAL**	**GRAFT LOST**
POS / NEG	10 [83.3%]	2 [16.7%]	15 [88.3%]	2 [11.7%]
NEG / POS	22 [75.8%]	7 [24.1%]	15 [88.3%]	2 [11.7%]
POS / POS	15 [71.4%]	6 [28.5%]	17 [77.3%]	5 [22.7%]
NEGATIVE SCREEN	233 [93.6%]	16 [6.4%]		

Table-4.9 shows presence of denovo HLA DSA and Non-DSA antibodies and graft survival. Antibody negative patients had better survival.

Graft survival

Study group graft outcome after six years patients who did not develop HLAab has better survival [93.6%], while those who develop de-novo DSA group had worst graft survival [83.3%], in further analysis DSA positive group, Class I DSA group had better survival than class II. In study group positive for both class I & II suffered the worst graft survival. In this study, we have discussed the detection of relevant antibody in kidney transplant. Below Kaplan-Meier graph-4.5 explain antibodies negative patients group has better survival then those who have develop post transplant antibody also Kaplan-Meier graph-4.6 shows development of denovo donor specific antibody(DSA) more harmful then non-DSA to the graft. Class -I antibodies are less harmful then class-II and presence of both class I & II shows poor outcome of transplant.

Detail has been already discussed earlier in this chapter. Graph 4.7 and Graph 4.8 explain how we are monitoring post transplant patients, in both graph we can see events time line like treatment given to patient, antibody level, S.Creatinine value for each patient.

GRAPH-4.5 Kaplan-Meierplot: **Negative vs DSA graft survival.**

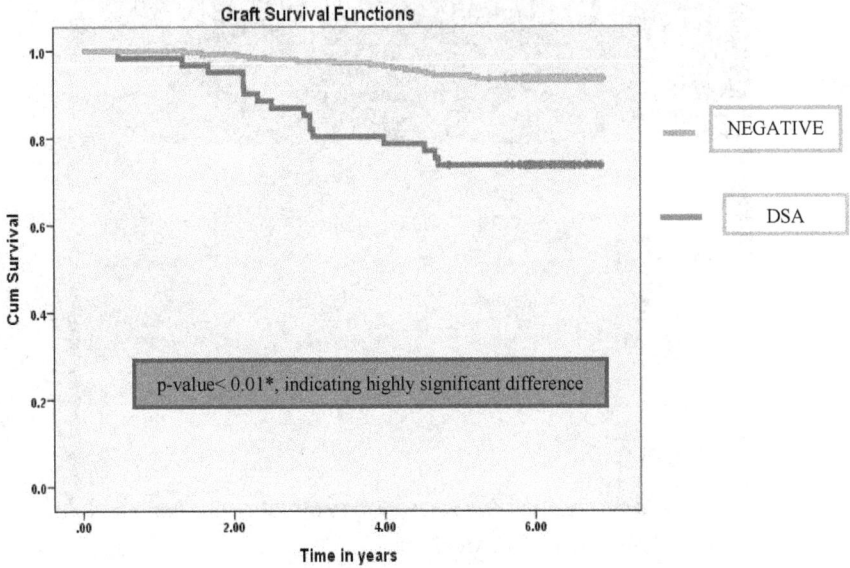

Graft Survival Functions

GRAPH-4.6 Kaplan-Meier**plot of DSA 1,DSA 1&2 and DSA 2**

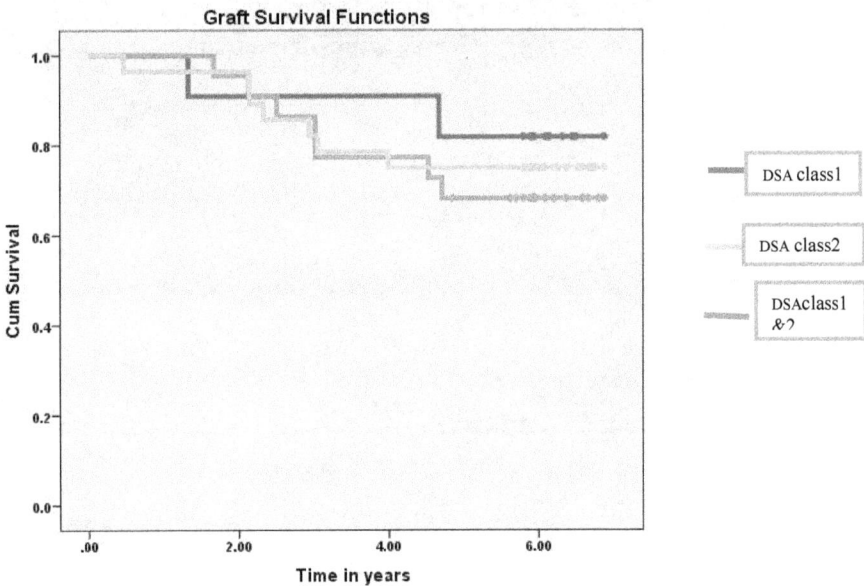

Graft Survival Functions

Graph-4.7 Post Transplant Monitoring

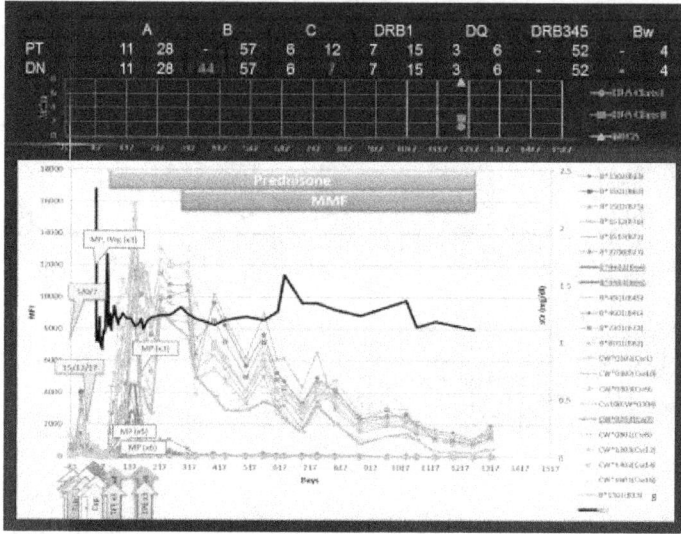

Graph-4.8 Post Transplant Monitoring

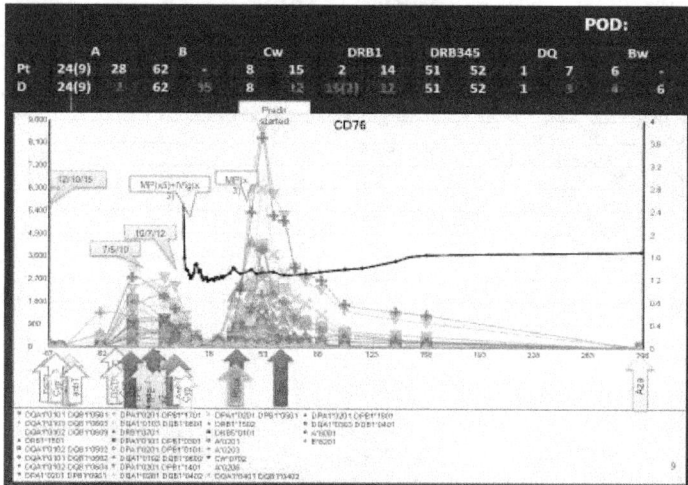

Above Two graphs explain post transplant follow-up
Top two rows show HLA typing of patient and donor, red colour HLA antigens are miss match antigens so antibody agnist this antigen called donor specific antibody (DSA)
X axis shows post transplant days.
Y axis shows single antigen bead assay in MFI
Arrow shows treatment given to patient at different point post-transplant
Black line indicates serum creatinine value
Bottom line indicates antibody specificities detected by single antigen test
Above both graphs explain that whenever there is HLA DSA antibodies kidney function remains unstable, with treatment (removal of antibody) graft remains stable

4.8 Rejection in kidney transplantation

Pathogenesis of acute and chronic renal allograft effects the survival. The antigenic targets, the mechanisms of T and B cell activation result in the production of antibody, the complement cascade, tests of antibody detection, and the indication that alloantibody-mediated mechanisms are active in acute and chronic rejection. T cell-mediated inflammation progressions in allograft rejection. To prevent and treat allograft rejection thus, have been directed against T cells. Developments of drugs have improved rates of acute cellular rejection and graft survival; acute rejection does occur, so as the long-term chronic rejection. The development of the immunohistochemical process for visualization of complement split product C4d in graft tissue that provided concrete evidence linking antibody binding and complement activation in renal allografts to the mechanism by which damage occurs in this setting (Feucht HE,1993). Alloantibodies play a role in rejections that do not respond to T cell therapies and, indeed, require targeted therapies that address the several mechanisms by which they exert their effects. More sensitive technologies for serum antibody screening are allowing for a clearer delineation of the relationship between antibodies and acute and chronic allograft pathologies and their attendant clinical outcomes. The antigenic targets of the humoral alloimmune response, the mechanism of antibody generation, the pathophysiology of antibody-mediated cell damage, the phenomenon of accommodation, and overview of the current understanding and classification of antibody-mediated syndromes, and the confirmation that antibodies are active in these clinical syndromes and the presently available therapies. It is essential that early regulatory responses leading to chronic rejection, at the time when interventions may alter the chronicity of graft injury remain to be defined. It is also important to categorize the acute allograft rejection.

The success of a renal transplant depends upon immunological and non-immunological reasons. Amongst immunological causes is allo-recognition through the allo-antigens. Alloantigen in the graft tissue is recognized by T cells in different forms. Monitoring for alloreactive memory T cells after organ transplantation allow individualization of immunosuppression. Two pathways of T cell allorecognition have been concerned in chronic graft dysfunction: Direct (recipient T cells respond to donor peptides presented by donor antigen-presenting cells) and indirect (donor peptides are processed and presented by recipient antigen-presenting cells). Complete allogeneic HLA molecules on the surface of donor tissue are able to directly activate T- cells; this is referred to as the direct pathway of allorecognition (Bestard et al. 2008). Direct pathway T cell activation is achieved by donor bone marrow-derived antigen-presenting cells; importantly, tissue dendritic cells migrate to draining lymphoid tissue soon after transplantation. The another pathway of MHC allorecognition is referred to as the 'indirect' pathway and includes the internalization, processing, and presentation of alloantigen as peptides bound to recipient MHC molecules. In the indirect pathway, T cells recognize donor allo-peptides on self-MHC molecules later being processed and presented by recipient APC.

Figure 4.1 Kidney TX: Strategies to prevent organ rejection

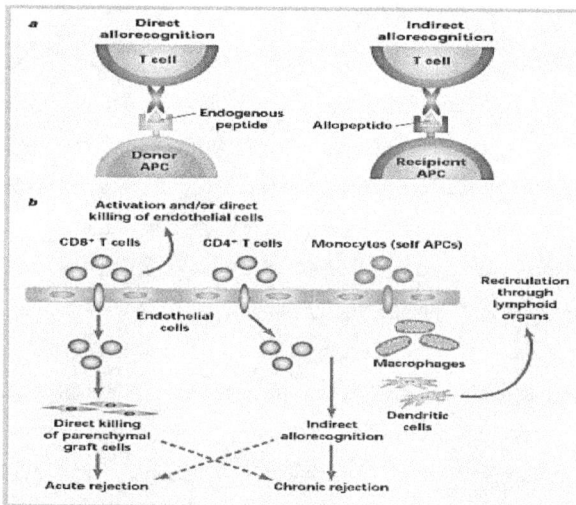

Role of HLA antigen matching on graft survival is a long-discussed issue, though; it has been shown that when the donor is MHC class II closely matched, a "hybrid" form of allorecognition (direct/indirect) occurs. The information of molecular immunology, better understanding of the methodologies to enhance graft survival is gaining acceptance and extensive use in human tissue and organ transplantation. The knowledge of molecular immunology, better understanding of the cellular and molecular mechanisms that highlight the immunological response to transplanted organ directed to the discovery of new immunosuppressive agents, such as tacrolimus, rapamycin, interleukin-2 receptor monoclonal antibodies, and mycophenolate mofetil. All these drugs show selective mechanisms for T and B cell alloimmune responses (Marina et al 2007). Currently combinations of various drugs are on trial and the results show that rejection rate has been reduced tremendously. Though, vigorous and prolonged immunosuppression results in infections and malignancies. If immune-tolerance can be established then side effects of immunosuppression can be reduced. The new generation drugs like FTY 20, antisense oligonucleotides are in the development. The trend is to develop agents, which are capable of blocking the co-stimulatory pathway of allorecognition so can result in tolerance (Haberala et al 2009).

Taken together, these collected discoveries have overthrown earlier concepts of the MHC class I and II regions as especially containing genes encoding for molecules which present antigenic peptides to T cells. Rather, the current view is a genetic region encoding different types of molecules collectively involved in pathways of antigen processing and presentation to helper and cytotoxic T cells. These gene products may have a role in immunologically mediated immune rejections (Zou et al 2009).

4.8.1 Mechanisms involved in allograft rejection

Immunological mechanisms involved in rejection could be (i) cell-mediated (ii) antibody-mediated

(i) T Cell-mediated Rejection

The allografts differ from the host at class I and class II loci. Both CD8+ and CD4+ T cells are activated by recognition of alloantigens of the grafts; the CD8+ T cells recognize foreign MHC class I molecules, which are expressed by all the cells in the graft. The differentiation of cytotoxic T lymphocytes (CTLs) is largely dependent on CD4+ T helper cells being stimulated by allogeneic class II molecules present on antigen-presenting cells (APCs) there are evidence, which suggest that some CD8+ T cells can also provide adequate help to allow cytotoxic T lymphocytes to differentiate independent of CD4+ T cells. Though, these CD8+ T cells appear to depend upon the professional APCs, like those required by conventional CD8+T cell. The most important APCs stimulating an antigraft response might be dendritic cells residing in the interstitium of the graft. Dendritic cells are regarded as critical instigators and regulators of immune reactivity, which play a role in both the direct and indirect pathways of allorecognition. Molecular signaling between dendritic cells and T cells directs the differentiation of naive (Th0) cells into either Th1 or Th2 cells.

(ii) Antibody-Mediated Rejection

The role of antibody in hyperacute rejection has been established (Singh et al 2009). A direct correlation is seen between positive pretransplant crossmatch which detects anti- MHC class I antibodies and the development of hyperacute rejection (Burns et al 2008). Anti-graft antibodies can be eluted from donor kidneys after hyperacute rejection. The passive transfer of antigraft antibodies in experimental models can aggravate hyperacute rejection. It is likely that antibodies also play a role in other types of rejection; though, their mechanisms remain incompletely understood and also controversial especially in chronic rejection (Burns et al 2008). The scanty cellular infiltrate in most cases of chronic rejection is antibody-mediated rejection. However, direct evidence for antibody-mediated damage in chronic dysfunction is inconclusive. The antibodies causing hyperacute rejection might be preformed (Hammer et al 1989) or they may develop under the influence of immunosuppressive drugs could modulate rate of production. Antibodies can bind to the graft, making the detection of soluble antigraft antibody difficult. Thus the role of antibody in the pathogenesis of chronic dysfunction remains undetermined. If immune-tolerance can be developed then side effects of immunosuppression can be reduced. The new generation drugs like FTY 20, antisense oligonucleotides are in the process of development. The trend is to develop agents, which are capable of blocking the co-stimulatory pathway of allorecognition which can result in tolerance (Haberala et al 2009).

4.8.2 Antibody Action without Complement

The action of antibody on endothelial cells in the absence of complement activation may have a role in allograft rejection, particularly chronic allograft rejection (Rahimi A, 1999). Even in the absence of complement, endothelial cells demonstrate activation and proliferation in the presence of MHC class I antibodies in vitro (Smith JD, 2000,Jin YP, 2002). This activation may be partly causative of arterial intimal proliferation that is characteristic of chronic humoral rejection. Noncomplement mechanisms, in the same way, may stem from direct antibody cell lysis through an Fc receptor on the surface of natural killer cells and macrophages; however, there is only limited evidence that this mechanism is related to acute rejection (Yuan FF, 2004).

4.8.3 Accommodation

Certain alloantibodies are not associated with acute graft injury and may correlate with good graft survival. The example of this is in long-term outcomes after ABO-incompatible transplantation. Despite that the anti-A/B antibodies return, the graft is not rejected (Tanabe K, 1998). The transient depletion of graft-specific antibodies at the time of transplantation prevents hyperacute rejection. If antibodies rebound within 10 days, then there is a high rate of acute rejection; however, if the antibody rebound is delayed until 3 weeks or later, then there is no correlation between titer and rejection. Such accommodation is formally defined as the resistance of an allograft to the acute pathologic effects of graft-specific antibodies and complement fixation (Koch CA, 2004). In HLA-mismatched grafts, the presence of alloantibodies in the absence of graft dysfunction criterion. It is clear that antibodies play an important role in the transplant outcome

4.9 Infection in transplant

Infectious complications a major cause of morbidity and mortality after kidney transplantation, particularly in the Asian population. Henceforth, prevention, early detection, and early treatment of such infections are crucial in kidney transplant recipients. Among all infectious complications, viruses are considered to be the common agents because of their abundance, infectivity, and latency ability. Herpes simplex virus, varicella-zoster virus, Epstein–Barr virus, cytomegalovirus, hepatitis B virus, BK polyomavirus, and adenovirus are well-known etiologic agents of viral infections in kidney transplant recipients worldwide for the reason that of their wide range of distribution. As DNA viruses, they can reactivate afterward affected patients receive immunosuppressive agents. These DNA viruses cause systemic diseases or allograft dysfunction, particularly in the first six months after transplantation. Pretransplant evaluation and immunization and appropriate prophylaxis and pre-emptive approaches after transplant have been recognized in the guidelines and are used to reduce the incidence of viral infections.

Although kidney transplantation is better than chronic dialysis, immunosuppression is a concern. There is an increased risk of infection in certain groups such as the elderly or undernourished people with chronic kidney diseases. The risk of infection increases further in patients in developing or tropical countries. In Thailand, the common causes of kidney recipient death are sepsis and pulmonary infection. In Asian countries, there is increased usage of potent immunosuppressive drugs as well as a transplant in high-risk patients, compared to the previous era of transplantation. Example, blood-group-incompatible kidney transplants require an aggressive preconditioning protocol; this approach particularly may result in cytomegalovirus (CMV) or BK polyomavirus (BKV) infection. CMV and BKV are the most common causes of viral infection after kidney transplantation. Though, clinical presentations vary; therefore, well-trained transplant physicians need to be conscious of this so that they can take care of the patients accordingly. Patients afflicted with CMV disease commonly present with fever, leucopenia, transaminitis, or enterocolitis. CMV disease is associated to high morbidity and mortality in transplant recipients. Preemptive treatment for CMV infection is recommended in CMV viremia, whereas preventive treatment is preferable in donor CMV immunoglobulin (Ig) G-positive and recipient IgG-negative (D+/ R−) cases [Fehr T, 2015, Kotton CN, 2010].

There has been an increased rate of viral infection observed in transplant patients. These infections are commonly acquired through dialysis or blood transfusion, especially viral hepatitis and human immunodeficiency virus (HIV). Thailand is an endemic area for the hepatitis A virus (HAV) and hepatitis B virus (HBV) [Sumethkul V, 2009, Lee J, 2016]. As a result, screening for these viruses in both potential donors and recipients be completed before transplantation. Donors with HBV or hepatitis C virus (HCV) handled with caution. Recipients immunized against HBV are allowed to have kidneys from HBV-infected donors; though, HB antibody level be carefully monitored [Chancharoenthana W, 2014]. Direct-acting antiviral (DAA) drugs have been developed. Though antiviral drugs against HBV remain an unfulfilled need, anti-HCV drugs are effective.

HIV is endemic in Thailand, and there are a substantial number of HIV-infected individuals with end-stage kidney disease. Due to their status, these individuals live with long-term dialysis and no opportunity for kidney transplantation. Although kidney transplantations in HIV-infected recipients have been widely performed in Western countries, immunosuppressive drugs are carefully prescribed [Locke JE, 2014]. Pretransplant evaluation requirement is carefully done, and post-transplant care for HIV-infected patients requires different attitudes. There is a strong drug-drug interaction between highly active antiretroviral therapy (HAART) and calcineurin inhibitors (CNIs); these drugs should be carefully used [Boyarsky BJ, 2015].

Posttransplant malignancy has been associated with many viral infections. Disturbing the immune system could lead to either allograft rejection or malignancy. Types of complications are associated with short graft and patient survival. Some viral infections are associated with the rejection of the graft or cause malignancy. Transplant physicians keep the patient's immune system in balance: too much immunosuppression might increase the risk of infection and malignancy, whereas too little immunosuppression could lead to rejection of the graft. Therefore, it is important to monitor the patient's health after transplantation to ensure that these complications do not occur.

4.9.1 General concept of viral infection in transplant recipients

Viruses are very small infectious agents that obligatory essential living host cells for replication. The viruses enter viable cells via attachment of viral proteins to specific receptors on the cell surface [Haywood AM, 1994]. Afterward the viruses have entered the host cells, they undergo viral replication. For RNA viruses, replication of the virus is completed in the cytoplasm of the host cell; and DNA viruses and retroviruses, replication of the virus occurs in the nucleus of the host cell. Discharging viral particles from the cells results in lysis of the cells; therefore, this process is termed the lytic phase [Traylen CM, 2011]. As soon as this phase occurs, viruses can spread to adjacent or distant uninfected cells via the bloodstream or neuronal route, causing viral illnesses [Knipe DM, 2001]. In immunocompetent individuals, viral infections are self-limiting because the intact innate (interferon [IFN]-α and β) and adaptive immunities (CD8+ cytotoxic T-lymphocyte, CD4+ helper T-cell subset) is capable of eliminating the viruses [Pang IK,2012, van de Berg PJ, 2008].

Some types of viruses can establish persistent infections in immunocompetent hosts, which can be divided into chronic and latent infections. Constant prolonged viral replication and shredding are observed in chronic viral infections (e.g., HBV and HCV), while maintenance of the viral genome without replication is found in latent viral infections (e.g., herpesviruses and polyomaviruses) [Chappell JD, 2015]. Latency is achieved once the genomes of the viruses remain in the nucleus or cytoplasm of the infected cells by subversion of the apoptotic pathways and not cleared by the host immune system [Randall RE, 2017, Kane M, 2010]. On the other hand, persistent host immune surveillance, especially by CD8+ T-cells and the persistent production of IFN-γ and tumor necrosis factor-α, are capable to block reactivation of latent infections [Khanna KM, 2004]. Receiving immunosuppressive agents following solid organ transplantation (SOT) can disturb the immune function and cause viral reactivation, mainly in the first six months after transplant [Humar A, 2006]. Some viruses, particularly CMV, have an indirect effect on the host immune system. Multiple proteins encoded by CMV contain immunomodulating activity that can either suppress the immune system or increase the inflammatory process. Hence, reactivation of CMV becomes an important risk factor in allograft rejection, as well as the acquisition of other opportunistic infections [Freeman RB, 2009]. CMV prophylaxis has been proven to help prevent CMV disease then in graft survival and overall outcomes [Roman A, 2014]. In adding to the direct and indirect effects of viral infection, it has been revealed that persistent viral infections can significantly increase the risk of malignancy among transplant recipients. Chronic inflammation and a failure to eliminate the pathogens contribute to viral oncogenesis. The reactions after the human immune system are supposed to be helpful for the host, but responses can too lead to DNA damage, aberrant cell proliferation, and neoangiogenesis. Oncogenic viruses can integrate into a host's genome and express their viral oncogenic protein [Carrillo-Infante C, 2007]. Some viruses may escape the host immune system by inducing the regulatory T-cells, which down-regulate the host immune response [Fehérvari Z, 2004]. The immunocompetent host, the immune system may control viral infection and check abnormal cell proliferation or neoangiogenesis processes. Unlike in the immunocompetent patient, though, patients on immunosuppressive medications (i.e., transplant recipients) have dysfunctional immune surveillance systems in immunosuppressed patients, cannot eradicate oncogenic viruses and premalignant cells.

Graph-4 viral infections in study group

Graph- 4.9 Viral Infection in Kidney Transplant.

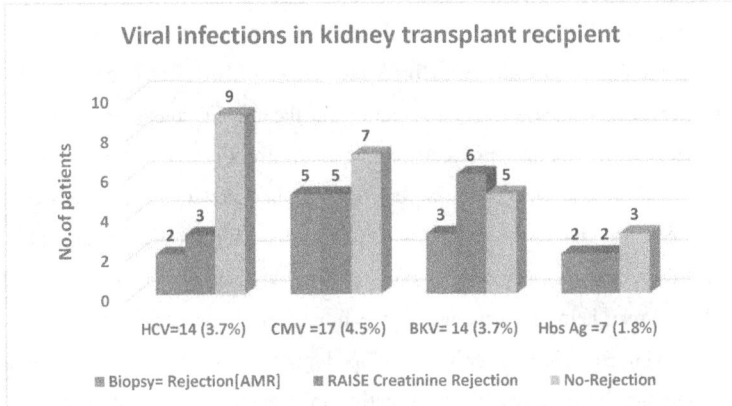

Graph shows infection, rejection and raise of serum creatinine during
Or after infection

Table-4.10 Viral infections in kidney transplant recipient

Infections	HCV=14	CMV =17	BKV= 14	Hbs Ag =7
%	3.7 %	4.5 %	3.7 %	1.8 %
Biopsy= Rejection[AMR]	2	5	3	2
RAISE Creatinine Rejection	3	5	6	2
No-Rejection	9	7	5	3

Table 4.10 shows rate of HCV (3.7%), CMV (4.5%), BKV (3.7%) and HBsAg (1.8%)
infections in post-transplant patients and rejection rate.

4.9.2 Common viral infection

We have found certain common viral infections in our study group, although the number of
infection was very few. Real analysis can be done including more number of patients. There is
no fix protocol for virus screening of transplant patients. Tests advice on the basis of history
and clinical symptoms and diagnosis.During this study one more paper published on BK virus
infection in post- transplantation (Trivedi v b 2019) BK virus (BKV) is a polyomavirus that

associated nephritis (BKVAN) and a significant risk factor for renal transplant dysfunction and allograft survival. The pathogenesis of BKVAN needs to be further investigated and the virus functions as still unclear; nevertheless there are a variety of hypotheses that indicate, host factors play important roles. Higher prevalence of BK virus infection in recent years has been correlated with acute rejection rates and the use of potent immunosuppressiveagents. Although over immunosuppression remains the primary risk factor for BK infection after transplantation, male gender, older recipient age and ureteral stent placement implicated as risk factors. The diagnosis of BKV is laboratory based method for its effects in urine, blood, and renal tissue. Some laboratory assay has provided new insights into the immune response to BK and may help guide therapy in the future. In the past, approximately 30% to 60% of patients with BK virus nephritis developed graft failure but early detection and routine screening has been shown to be effective in preventing allograft loss. In the study, we screened 1240 patients and out of these 106 (8.54%) found positive for BKV. The rate of viruria and viremia were 69 (65%) and 37 (34.9%) out of total BKV positive. Their mean of serum creatinine level were 1.56±0.2 mg/dl and 2.39 ± 0.3 mg/dl in viruria and viremia, respectively.

Table-4.11 study group viruria vs viremia Total 1240 patients were tested.

GROUP= Total 106 Patients positive 106 (8.54%)	VIRURIA= 69 Patients (65%)	VIREMIA = 37 Patients (34.9%)
SEX	57 M + 12 F	34 M/ 3 F
MEAN S. Creatinine	1.56±0.2 mg/dl	2.39 ± 0.3 mg dl
Average BKV Positive to Negative period	274 Days	112 Days
Lost Follow-up	16 [2BK+14 AMR]	9 [3 BK+6AMR]
Allograft Loss	5	4
Patients Loss	1	2

Table 4.11shows male/female ratio mean, S.Creatinine mg/dl, Infection clearing in days, lost to follow up patients, graft lost and patients lost, number of patients with viruria and viremia

Table-4.12 HLA match VS BK infection virus found in blood (VIREMIA)

GROUP-1 VIREMIA = 37 Patients HLA MATCH A,B,Cw,DR,DQ	PT's	LOST FOLLOW	Allograft LOSS	REJ. S.Creatinine	REJ. Graft Biopsy	2013	2014	2015	2016	2017
0	6			3	1 AMR					
1	4			2	2 AMR					
2	5	1	1	1	1 BK[exp]			1	1	
3	5	2		3		1	1			
4	4	2	1	4			1		1	1
5	10	4	2	3	2 BK + 3 AMR [1 exp]		1	4	1	1
6	2			2						
7	1			0						

Table 4.12 shows in detail number of patients suffered rejections, HLA match and infection, lost to follow up, Graft lost in viremia group.

Table-4.13 HLA match VS BK infection virus found in urine (VIRURIA)

GROUP-2 VIRURIA= 69 Patients HLA MATCH A,B,Cw,DR,DQ	PT's	LOST FOLLOW	Allograft LOSS	REJ. S.Creatinine	REJ. Graft Biopsy	2013	2014	2015	2016	2017
0	24	4	3	7	2 AMR	2	1 + 1	1 + 1	3 + 1	
1	2	1		1					1	
2	8	1		2	2 AMR			1		
3	6	2	1	3	3 AMR	1	1	1		
4	5	2	1	2	2 AMR			1	1	1
5	19	3		6	2 BK+ 8 AMR	2	1			
6	2	2		1	1 AMR		1	1		
7	2	1						1		
8	1									

Table 4.13 shows in detail number of patients suffered rejections, HLA match and infection, lost to follow up, Graft lost in viruria group.

We obtained some important data about BKV infection, that early diagnosis of viruriaand viremia, immunosuppression reduction and use of antiviral therapy or the combination of both are BKV nephropathy treatment and management options.

Chapter - 5

Summary & Scope

Chapter - 5

Summary and scope of the study:

The main aim of this study is to address following questions: 1) How to improve graft survival by closely monitoring patients, 2) How to deal with the problem of rejection and infection (protocol for regular testing), and 3) How to increase the number of the transplant by innovative approach (swap donor).

In our study, total370 patients consecutively transplanted were enrolled and studied for five years. Out of which 312 patients received a kidney from living related donor while 58 patients received a kidney from swap donor. Transplanted graft outcome in both groups was comparable.

All patients and donors were HLA typed for HLA A, B, C, DR and DQ antigens and different types of crossmatches were performed like Auto, CDC, FCM T & B cell, and single antigen.All crossmatches information was analyzed on the basis of patient's history, sensitivity and specificity of tests to know relevance ofidentified antibodies and immunological risk involvedin transplantation. Post-transplant period specifically looking for HLA (class I and II) antibodywhichcauses acute and chronic rejection. In Asian countries, there is a problem of infections in the post-transplant period because of immunosuppression drugs. Therefore, all patients were monitored for infection and development of donor-specific antibody (DSA) against HLA class I & II mismatched antigens. In India, kidney transplant for ESRD patients is very expensive and also not getting support from society particularly for female patients. Most of the transplant carried out are living related donor. Unrelated living donor transplant are illegal so it is hard to find a healthy voluntary donor from family so there is a great need to increase donor pool, for that we have to come up with novel ideas. At IKDRC, (I) swap donor transplant is offered since seven years. Patient-donor can be a one-way swap or long-chain to find best match patient and donor pair. Transplant outcome is equally good compare to other living donors. (II) The second type is ABO-incompatible transplant where the living donor is a mismatch for the ABO blood group. Criteria for organ donation is same as blood group donation but Rh group matching not required. There are more chances of infection because a patient is more immunosuppressed. This method is very expensive not so popular in India. (III) The third one is Expanded Criteria Donor (ECD) donor old age more than 60 years in our scenario more than 50% of donors were parents or disease donor in both group donor is meeting ECD guidelines

89

than organ is accepted for donation. (IV) The fourth one is swap donor in which mismatch blood group, the age difference between patient and donor and sensitized patients who already have a living related donor but crossmatch is positive, so considering antibody profile crossmatch negative donor can be found for this group of patients. In post-transplant period all patients were monitored for donor-specific antibody (DSA) as per protocol 1, 3, 6 monthly and then yearly; if meanwhile recipient develop DSA HLA antibody, then they are more prone to acute or chronic rejection; thus the appearance of DSA post-transplant is bad news and patient is treated to remove those antibodies with IVIG, plasmapheresis and Bortezomib, optimization of immunosuppression medication and closely monitoring for DSA and infections. Alloantibody, either preexisting or de novo developed, are associated with hyperacute, acute, and chronic rejection. Post-transplantation antibody monitoring becomes extremely critical in transplant clinics, not only because it can help to determine the extent of a patient's humoral response to allograft but also, and perhaps more importantly, it will direct clinicians to optimize immunosuppressive therapy. In HLA Mismatch Immunogenicity mismatched HLA antigens have different epitope "loads". HLA epitopes have different degrees of immunogenicity. A better understanding of HLA immunogenicity will permit a permissible mismatch strategy for non-sensitized transplant patients.

The important finding from this study reveals that most of the centers considering HLA A, B and DR antigen for match and graft survival but the role of de novo DQ antibody was not clear. Our study Data shows 24.3 % patients develop de novo DSA out of that 45.8 % were DQ only or added class-I or DR antibodies. Those who had DQ DSA with more than 10,000 MFI had rapid progressive graft failure (18.5%) than less than 5000 MFI, over five years. This study discusses factors affecting long-term graft survival in kidney transplant patients and also need for preventive, prophylactic and surveillance testing for infection.

Scope for future study

Different transplant immunology centers in the world are doing research how to block immunological activity which harms transplanted kidney and also try to find best matching donor so that in a post-transplant period there is less immunological responses activity or to create tolerance. Virtual crossmatch (VXM) analysis involved serological and epitope identification. The serological analysis matched the serological HLA typing and antibody detection to detect the serological donor-specific antibody (sDSA). The highest MFI value was recorded if over one bead was positive for the same antigen. In cases of multiple DSA, both the total and the peak DSA MFI are recorded. The epitope analysis performed by HLA-Matchmaker version 02.0 for HLA-ABC, and version 02.1 for HLA-DR, HLA-DQ, and HLA-DP (*https://www.epitopes.net*). HLA-Matchmaker is a structurally based computer algorithm that can determine HLA matching at epitope level. This method was able to determine both verified and unverified eplets. The MFI of the immunized eplet was recorded. In cases of multiple DSA, both the total and the peak of the DSA MFI were recorded. Researches are trying to establish the detrimental effect of complement fixing antibodies on graft survival. For this, test is carried out is C1q on Luminex platform. Other research going on Non-HLA antigen and Autoantibodies. Antibodies that are specific to organ donor HLA have been involved in the most of cases of antibody-mediated rejection in solid organ transplant recipients. Though, recent data show that production of non-HLA autoantibodies can occur before transplant in the form of natural autoantibodies. While HLAs are constitutively expressed on the cell surface of the allograft endothelium, autoantigens are generally cryptic. Tissue damage associated with ischemia-reperfusion, vascular injury, and/or rejection creates permissive situations for the expression of cryptic autoantigens, allowing these autoantibodies to bind antigenic targets and further enhance vascular inflammation and renal dysfunction. Anti-perlecan/LG3 antibodies and anti-angiotensin II type 1 receptor antibodies have been found before transplant or de novo transplants indicate negative long–term outcome in patients with renal transplants. Evidence suggesting a significant role for autoantibodies to cryptic antigens as novel accelerators of kidney dysfunction and acute or chronic allograft rejection.

Though infections continue to play a significant role in morbidity and mortality after transplantation, better prophylactic, diagnostic, and treatment strategies have decreased the negative effect of infection on transplant outcomes. Ongoing care to infection prevention beginning before transplantation, as well as enhanced surveillance for infections, must be maintained in all patients being considered for transplantation.

9 783054 827922